Department of Veterans Affairs
Health Services Research & Development Service

Evidence Synthesis Pilot Program

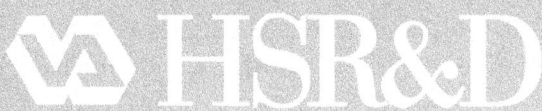

I0470835

Screening Men for Osteoporosis: Who & How

May 2007

Prepared for:

Department of Veterans Affairs
Veterans Health Administration
Health Services Research & Development Service
Washington, DC 20420

Prepared by:

Greater Los Angeles Veterans Affairs Healthcare
System/Southern California/RAND Evidence-based
Practice Center
Los Angeles, CA

Investigators:

Paul Shekelle, MD, PhD
Director

Brett Munjas, BA
Project Manager/Literature Database Manager

Hau Liu, MD
Elaine Wong, MD
Content Experts/Physician Reviewers

Neil Paige, MD
Caroline Goldzweig, MD
Physician Reviewers/Health Services Researchers

Annie Zhou, MS
Marika Suttorp, MS
Statisticians

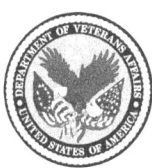

Suggested Citation

Shekelle P, Munjas B, Liu H, Paige N, and Zhou A. "Screening Men for Osteoporosis: Who & How." Department of Veterans Affairs. May 2007.

Technical Experts & Consultants*

Eric Orwoll, MD, Oregon Health Sciences University, Portland, OR.

William Duncan, MD, VA Central Office, Washington, DC.

Service as a technical expert for this report does not imply endorsement of the report's findings.

FINANCIAL DISCLOSURE: No investigators have any affiliations or financial involvement (e.g., employment, consultancies, honoraria, stock ownership or options, expert testimony, grants or patents received or pending, or royalties) that conflict with material presented in the report.

PREFACE

VA's Health Services Research and Development Service (HSR&D) works to improve the cost, quality, and outcomes of health care for our nation's veterans. Collaborating with VA leaders, managers, and policy makers, HSR&D focuses on important health care topics that are likely to have significant impact on quality improvement efforts. One significant collaborative effort is HSR&D's Evidence-based Synthesis Pilot Project (ESP). Through this project, HSR&D provides timely and accurate evidence syntheses on targeted health care topics. These products will be disseminated broadly throughout VA and will: inform VA clinical policy, develop clinical practice guidelines, set directions for future research to address gaps in knowledge, identify the evidence to support VA performance measures, and rationalize drug formulary decisions.

HSR&D provided funding for the two Evidence Based Practice Centers (EPCs) supported by the Agency for Healthcare Research and Quality (AHRQ) that also had an active and publicly acknowledged VA affiliation—Southern California EPC and Portland, OR EPC—so they could develop evidence syntheses on requested topics for dissemination to VA policymakers. A planning committee with representation from HSR&D, Patient Care Services, Office of Quality and Performance, and the VISN Clinical Management Officers, has been established to identify priority topics and to insure the quality of final reports.

Comments on this evidence report are welcome and can be sent to Susan Schiffner, ESP Program Manager, at Susan.Schiffner@va.gov .

TABLE OF CONTENTS

FIGURES

APPENDIX

Appendix A. Data Collection Forms
Appendix B. Evidence Table

EXECUTIVE SUMMARY

BACKGROUND

Although 25% of men over the age of 60 will sustain osteoporotic fractures during their lifetime, data suggest that male osteoporosis is underdiganosed and undertreated. In order to help inform decisions about whether the Veterans Health Administration should develop screening guidelines for male osteoporosis, summaries of what is known about 1) the epidemiology of male osteoporosis, and 2) the validity of tools to screen and diagnose male osteoporosis are needed.

The Key Questions were:

Key Question 1. What are the prevalence of and risk factors for osteopenia, osteoporosis and osteoporotic fractures among men in general and among male Veterans specifically?

Key Question 2. Are there any validated tools (outside of central bone density) to screen for osteoporosis in men?

Key Question 3. What values of BMD determined by Dual energy X-ray Absorptiometry (DXA) (and by different DXA techniques) have been used to diagnose osteopenia and osteoporosis; and what is the evidence regarding the relationship between differing definitions and the development of osteoporotic fractures?

METHODS

We searched PubMed from 1990-2006 using standard search terms. Titles, abstracts, and articles were reviewed in duplicate by physicians trained in the critical analysis of literature. Data were extracted by quantitative analysts. Pooled analyses were performed for the comparison of either calcaneal ultrasound or the Osteoporosis Screening Tool compared to central DXA; all other data were narratively summarized.

RESULTS

We screened 564 titles and performed a more detailed review on 378 articles. From this, we identified 173 articles that addressed risk factors for osteoporosis, 27 articles that addressed diagnostic tools, and 31 articles about differing DXA levels and fracture risk. We identified an older high quality meta-analysis of risk factors for osteoporosis. Of the risk factors assessed in this review that the authors classified as something other than high risk, VA policymakers selected alcohol use, diabetes mellitus type II, and spinal cord injury as the factors for assessment in this review.

KEY QUESTION #1: What are the prevalence of and risk factors for osteopenia, osteoporosis and osteoporotic fractures among men in general and among male Veterans specifically?

PREVALENCE

- There are no VA specific data on prevalence of osteopenia and osteoporosis in men.
- Applying NHANES III estimates of prevalence to veteran-specific enrollee data we estimate the prevalence of osteoporosis in male veterans of 200,000 – 400,000; and of osteopenia in male veterans of 2-3 million.

RISK FACTORS

- We found a high quality meta-analysis, and a limited number of articles specific to the risk factors alcohol use, diabetes mellitus type II and spinal cord injury. Based on these findings, our review suggests the following.
- Strong predictors of an increased risk of osteoporosis in men include age, low body weight, physical inactivity, and weight loss. (GRADE quality of evidence = High; further research is very unlikely to change our confidence on the estimate of effect.)
- Certain health conditions and medications also are strong or moderate predictors of an increased risk of osteoporosis in men. The most relevant to VA are prolonged systemic corticosteroid therapy and androgen deprivation (in the context of prostate cancer treatment). (GRADE quality of evidence = Moderate; further research is likely to have an important impact on our confidence in the estimate of effect and may change the estimate.)
- Alcohol use is probably associated with an increase in osteoporotic fractures, but is not clearly associated with an increase in osteoporosis as measured by BMD. (GRADE quality of evidence: Fractures = Moderate; further research is likely to have an important impact on our confidence in the estimate of effect and may change the estimate; BMD = Very Low; any estimate of effect is very uncertain.)
- There is no evidence that diabetes mellitus type II is a significant risk factor for osteoporosis in men. (GRADE quality of evidence: Low; further research is very likely to have an important impact on our confidence in the estimate of effect and is likely to change the estimate.)
- Spinal Cord Injury is likely associated with an increase risk of osteoporosis and possibly osteoporotic fractures. (GRADE quality of evidence: BMD=Moderate; further research is likely to have an important impact on our confidence in the estimate of effect and may change the estimate; Fractures=Low; further research is very likely to have an important impact on our confidence in the estimate of effect and is likely to change the estimate.)

KEY QUESTION #2: Are there any validated tools (outside of central bone density) to screen for osteoporosis in men?

- The evidence for screening tools for men is much more limited than for women. We were only able to synthesize evidence on two screening tools: calcaneal ultrasound and the Osteoporosis Screening Tool (OST).
- There is no evidence to suggest that calcaneal ultrasound performs differently in men than in women. (GRADE quality of evidence = Moderate; further research is likely to have an important impact on our confidence in the estimate of effect and may change the estimate.)

- The OST appears to have comparable (and possibly better) test characteristics than calcaneal ultrasound in diagnosing DXA-determined osteoporosis. (GRADE quality of evidence = Low; further research is very likely to have an important impact on our confidence in the estimate of effect and is likely to change the estimate.)
- Although calcaneal ultrasound does not appear to be a particularly good test at diagnosing DXA-determined osteoporosis, it is a strong, independent predictor of fractures in men. (GRADE quality of evidence = Moderate; further research is likely to have an important impact on our confidence in the estimate of effect and may change the estimate.)
- Limited data are available on other screening modalities and there is a large gap in our understanding of osteoporosis screening tests in men.

KEY QUESTION #3: What values of BMD determined by DXA (and by different DXA techniques) have been used to diagnose osteopenia and osteoporosis; and what is the evidence regarding the relationship between differing definitions and the development of osteoporotic fractures?

- The values of BMD determined by DXA that have been used are based on standard deviations (T-score) away from a reference standard, either young female or young male.
- Whether to use a young female or a young male reference range in order to identify men as "at risk" for osteoporotic fractures is an area of controversy that is not possible to resolve with existing data.
- Until more definitive evidence is available, we believe it is most logically consistent for VA to use for the identification of men who might potentially benefit from treatment for osteoporosis the same conditions as were used in the randomized controlled trials (RCT), in other words use of the young male reference standard. (GRADE quality of evidence = Low; further research is very likely to have an important impact on our confidence in the estimate of effect and is likely to change the estimate.)

INTRODUCTION

Background

Although the Surgeon General's recent report on osteoporosis stated that, "Strong bones (are) essential to overall health and quality of life," it warned that, "The bone health status of Americans... is in jeopardy."[1] Traditionally, osteoporosis was viewed as a disease of women, but it has become clear that osteoporotic fractures result in substantial morbidity, mortality, and costs in men.[2-6] A 60-year old man has a 25% lifetime risk of sustaining an osteoporotic fracture.[7] The consequences of this fracture can be severe as the one-year mortality rate in men after hip fracture is twice that of women.[8] With the aging of the population, rates of osteoporosis in men are expected to increase nearly 50% in the next 15 years and hip fractures rates are projected to double or triple by 2040.[1]

Furthermore, annual U.S. direct medical costs for osteoporosis exceed $17 billion[9] and are expected to increase rapidly with an aging population.[1] The percentage of costs directly attributable to men or veterans is unclear, although 25% of hip fractures, the fracture type associated with greatest costs due to hospitalization and long-term care, occur in men.[5] This large and growing clinical and cost burden, combined with an environment of increasingly limited health care resources, strongly underlies the need to develop rational, evidence-based osteoporosis management strategies to obtain maximum benefit for every health care dollar spent.

Osteoporotic fractures may be particularly devastating in the veteran population as post-fracture inpatient mortality rates for Veterans are more than double that of the general population.[10] An analysis of femoral bone mineral density data from the National Health and Nutrition Examination Survey (NHANES) III, a nationally-representative dataset, reported that 1 to 2 million American men over the age of 50 have osteoporosis and 8 to 13 million similarly-aged men have osteopenia, or low bone density.[11] Applying prevalence data from this analysis to VA-specific enrollee data,[12] it is possible that 200,000 to 400,000 veterans have osteoporosis and 2 to 3 million veterans have osteopenia. These estimates are likely conservative as Veterans have increased rates of co-morbid conditions compared to the general population.[13]

Despite the substantial advances in our understanding of osteoporosis over the last decade, there are no consensus guidelines on the assessment and management of male osteoporosis. Although osteoporosis management strategies have been evaluated in women,[1,14-19] much less work has been done in this area in men.[10,20,21] Lack of research in this area has led to considerable uncertainty regarding optimal osteoporosis strategies in men and Veterans. The VA Office of Quality and Performance and the U.S. Preventive Services Task Force offer no clinical practice guidelines on the management of osteoporosis in men. The National Osteoporosis Foundation offers no guidelines on screening for men, although it suggests that that all individuals be treated with osteoporosis medications if they have a pre-existing fragility fracture.[22] The International Society for Clinical Densitometry suggests that all men over the age of 70 receive a DXA exam,[23] although the effects of this recommendation have not been evaluated. As such, a significant gap in our understanding exists on how best to evaluate and manage osteoporosis in men.

As the largest integrated health care system in the U.S., serving a population that is more than 95% male and 80% over the age of 50,[12] these issues are of particular concern and importance to the VA. In particular, identifying and implementing optimal strategies for osteoporosis management will be critically important over the next five to ten years as the "baby boomers" begin to reach retirement, an age when fracture risk dramatically increases in men. Given the large number of male veterans at high risk for osteoporosis who receive care through the VA, the VA is uniquely positioned and qualified to dramatically preserve and improve veteran and male skeletal health

In order to inform decision-making regarding potential VA screening guidelines for male osteoporosis, William Duncan, MD, PhD, the Acting Director of the VA Medical Service, and the VA HSR&D Service commissioned this literature review of the epidemiology and risk factors for osteoporosis, and validity of screening tools for male osteoporosis. This review is being performed as part of the Evidence Synthesis Project, an HSR&D-organized initiative to provide VA policymakers with high quality evidence reviews.

The purpose of this review is to analyze the literature in order to answer three key questions: 1) What is the epidemiology and what are the key risk factors for male osteoporosis?; 2) Are there any validated screening tools for osteoporosis in men (beyond DXA-assessed central bone density)?; and 3) What is the evidence regarding bone mineral density and fracture risk? The results of this review will be used to assist VA policy-makers in making evidence-based decisions on how best to preserve and improve skeletal health in the veteran population. In specific, their report is not meant to be a guideline. The role of guideline development is that of the VA guidelines committee, which will use this evidence synthesis in its deliberation.

METHODS

Topic Development

This project was nominated by William Duncan, MD, for the Evidence Synthesis Project. Key questions were discussed and finalized during a conference call that included the Steering Committee of the Evidence Synthesis Project, Dr. Duncan, and the VA Greater Los Angeles project site director. The final key questions are:

1. What are the prevalence of and risk factors for osteopenia, osteoporosis and osteoporotic fractures among men in general and among male Veterans specifically?

2. Are there any validated tools (outside of central bone density) to screen for osteoporosis in men?

3. What values of BMD determined by DXA (and by different DXA techniques) have been used to diagnose osteopenia and osteoporosis; and what is the evidence regarding the relationship between differing definitions and the development of osteoporotic fractures?

Search Strategy

Our library searches began in June, 2006, with a search of PubMed.

The search strategy is listed below:

DATABASE SEARCHED & TIME PERIOD COVERED:
 PUBMED – 1990-2006

LIMITERS: ENGLISH, HUMAN, MALE

SEARCH STRATEGY:
osteoporosis[majr] OR osteoporosis[ti]
AND
male[tiab] OR men[tiab] OR gender
AND
risk factors[majr] OR risk*[tiab]
AND
bone mineral density OR bone*[ti] OR risk*[ti] OR fractur*[ti]
NOT
Results of previous searches

NUMBER OF ITEMS RETRIEVED: 508

In addition to our PubMed search, we performed reference mining of retrieved articles, references of prior reviews, and solicited articles from experts.

Study Selection

Four trained researchers (working in groups of two) reviewed the list of titles and selected articles for further review. Each group of two consisted of an endocrinologist trained in the critical examination of literature and a fellowship-trained health services research general internist. Each article retrieved was reviewed with a brief screening form (see Appendix A) that collected data on prevalence and incidence, risk fractures, diagnostic tools, associations between bone mass density levels (BMD) as determined by dual energy X-ray absorptiometry (DXA), study design, and whether or not the subjects in the study were Veterans. To be included in our evidence report, a study had to measure incidence, prevalence, or risk factors for osteoporosis in men; or, a comparison of two different methods of assessing for the presence of osteoporosis in men; or, provide data on different values of BMD as determined by DXA and risk of osteoporotic fractures in men. Eligible study designs included controlled clinical trials, cohort studies and case series, case control studies, and systematic reviews/meta-analyses. Case reports, non-systematic reviews, letters to the editor and other similar contributions were excluded.

Data Abstraction

Data were independently abstracted by an endocrinologist and a general internist/health services researcher, with consensus resolution. The following data were abstracted from included trials: study test and site, reference test and site, population, sample size, patient characteristics, region, and outcome reporting. Data abstraction forms are provided in Appendix A.

For diagnostic accuracy studies, a statistician extracted data. For each selected study, the sample size, sensitivity and specificity at each quantitative ultrasound or questionnaire threshold were extracted. The standard error of sensitivity and specificity were calculated as $variance_{sens} = p_i*(1-p_i)/n_i$ where p_i is the sensitivity for study i and n_i is the number of people classified as having the disease for study i. If a study did not report the sensitivity or specificity and if they could not be calculated from the given data, the study was excluded from analysis. We contacted the original authors of some studies to obtain the sample sizes per group needed to perform this calculation.

Quality assessment

To assess internal validity of diagnostic studies, we used the QUADAS, a tool for Quality Assessment of studies of Diagnostic Accuracy included in Systematic Reviews (see Appendix A). We abstracted data on representativeness of patients to those who will receive the test in practice; clarity of selection criteria; likelihood of reference test to correctly classify the condition; time frame between reference test and study test; whether or not the entire or randomized group of the sample received verification using the reference test; whether patients received the same reference test regardless of the study test result; independence of the reference test from the study test; ability to replicate study and reference test based on detail provided in the article; study test results interpreted blinded from reference standard and vice versa; replicability of results when test is used in practice; and whether intermediate test results were reported; withdrawals from the study explained.

To assess internal validity of studies of risk or prognosis, we used the criteria proposed by Hayden and colleagues[24] (see Appendix A). We abstracted data on study participation; study attrition, prognostic factor measurement; outcome measurement; confounding measurement and account; and analysis.

Rating the body of evidence

We assessed the overall quality of evidence for outcomes using a method developed by the Grade Working Group, which classified the grade of evidence across outcomes according to the following criteria:[25]

- o **High** = Further research is very unlikely to change our confidence on the estimate of effect.
- o **Moderate** = Further research is likely to have an important impact on our confidence in the estimate of effect and may change the estimate.
- o **Low** = Further research is very likely to have an important impact on our confidence in the estimate of effect and is likely to change the estimate.
- o **Very Low** = Any estimate of effect is very uncertain.

GRADE also suggests using the following scheme for assigning the "grade" or strength of evidence:

Criteria for assigning grade of evidence
Type of evidence
Randomized trial = high
Observational study = low
Any other evidence = very low
Decrease grade if:
• Serious (-1) or very serious (-2) limitation to study quality
• Important inconsistency (-1)
• Some (-1) or major (-2) uncertainty about directness
• Imprecise or sparse data (-1)
• High probability of reporting bias (-1)
Increase grade if:
• Strong evidence of association-significant relative risk of > 2 (< 0.5) based on consistent evidence from two or more observational studies, with no plausible confounders (+1)
• Very strong evidence of association-significant relative risk of > 5 (< 0.2) based on direct evidence with no major threats to validity (+2)
• Evidence of a dose response gradient (+1)
• All plausible confounders would have reduced the effect (+1)

For this report, we used both this explicit scoring scheme and the global implicit judgment about "confidence" in the result. Where the two disagreed, we went with the lower of the two classifications.

Data Synthesis

Of the articles that were determined to be clinically eligible, thresholds for determining osteoporosis (in terms of T-scores) were reviewed across studies to see if they were comparable. First, we looked to see if the diagnostic method used was similar across studies. Then, within diagnostic method, we looked to see if the cutoff points analyzed were consistent across studies. Within comparable measures, we estimated a pooled random effects estimate[26] of the sensitivity and specificity. ROC (receiver operating characteristic) curves were graphed. Pooled estimates from the meta analysis were plotted onto the ROC curves.

The remaining studies regarding diagnostic assessments were too heterogeneous to statistically pool, and we therefore summarized these narratively.

Peer Review

This report was reviewed by our technical experts. Their comments were taken into consideration in our revision. Service as a technical expert does not imply endorsement of the report's findings.

RESULTS

Literature Flow

In total, we examined 580 titles. The electronic literature search identified 508 articles. An additional 68 articles were identified through reference mining. Content experts identified 4 more articles.

Of the titles identified through our electronic literature search, 186 were rejected as not relevant to the project. This left 394 from all sources. Four articles were excluded at abstract review. One title could not be located after contacting many sources.

Initial screening of the articles resulted in 176 articles that addressed risk factors for osteoporosis. We found 27 articles that addressed diagnostic tools for osteoporosis, and 31 articles about differing DXA levels and risk of fracture. (Figure 1)

Figure 1. Male OP Literature Flow

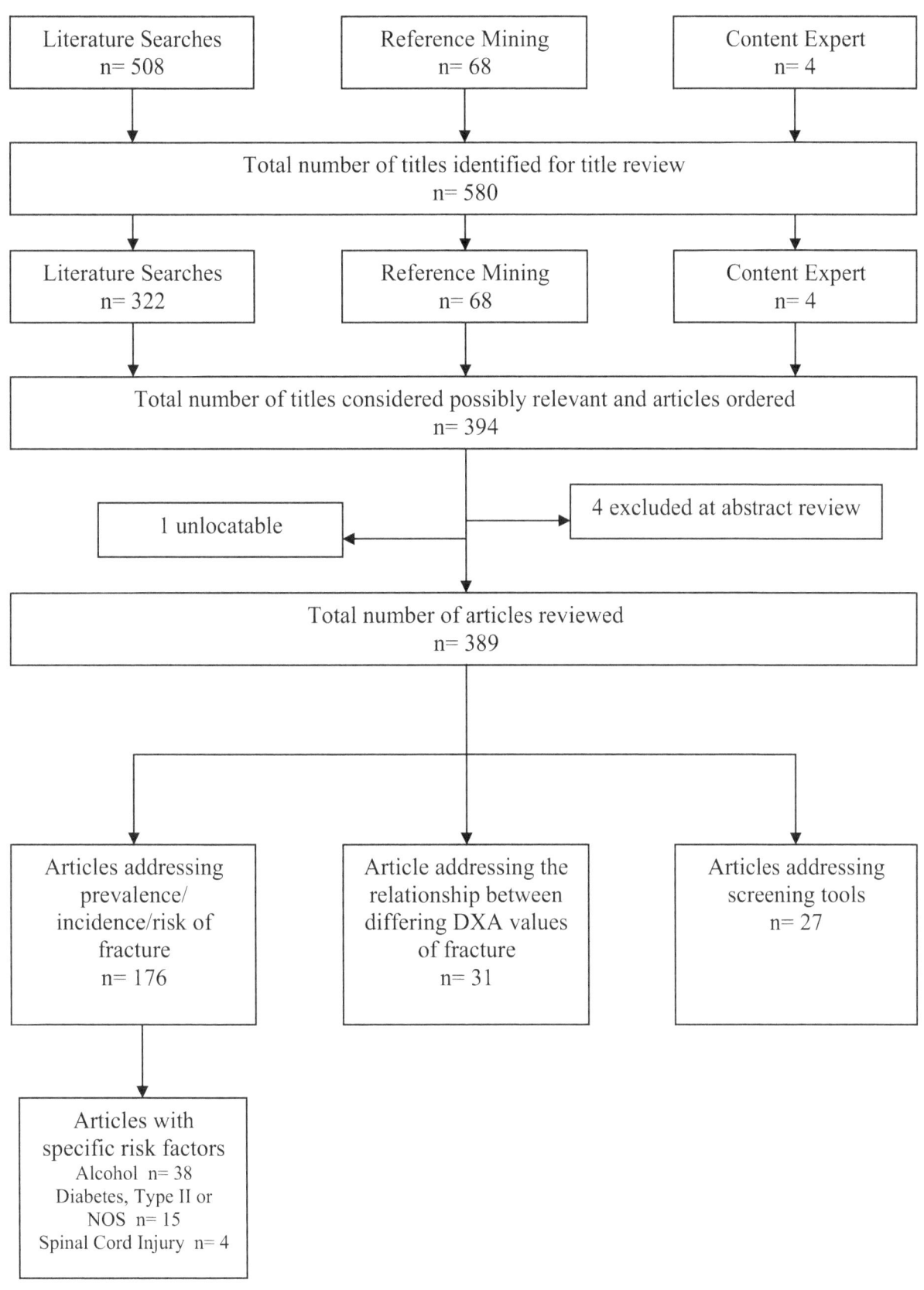

Key Question #1: What are the prevalence of and risk factors for osteopenia, osteoporosis and osteoporotic fractures among men in general and among male Veterans specifically?

PREVALENCE

We identified 20 articles that compared osteoporosis and men in Veteran populations.[10,19,27-44] All of the articles dealt with patients selected from specific populations such as nursing homes, pulmonary clinic, rheumatology clinic, etc.; or, were convenience samples. Thus there are no population-based data on the prevalence of osteoporosis in male veterans.

A study assessing the prevalence of osteoporosis using a T-score of >2.5 standard deviations below the young male reference standard, based on data from the National Health and Nutrition Examination Survey III (NHANES III), estimated that the prevalence in men was 3%-6% for osteoporosis, and 28%-27% for osteopenia.[11] Applying these estimates of prevalence to VA-specific enrollee data yields estimates of 200,000 to 400,000 male veterans with osteoporosis and 2 to 3 million male veterans with osteopenia.

RISK FACTORS

We identified a high quality systematic review and meta-analysis seeking to identify factors to help select subjects for bone densitometry assessments.[45] This review searched multiple computerized databases up to 1997 and identified 94 cohort studies, 72 case control studies, and 1 randomized clinical trial. Most studies were performed in subjects older than age 50 and used American or European populations. Where feasible, the authors used fixed-effects methods to provide meta-analytic pooled estimates of risk. They classified risk factors into the following groups:

"High risk": an associated Relative Risk (RR) or Odds Ratio (OR) of greater than or equal to 2.
"Moderate risk": risk vales of between 1 and 2.
"No risk": risk values close to or equal to the null value, or even a protective effect.
"Unclassifiable": the data are insufficient or contradictory to reach a conclusion.

The authors performed separate analyses for men and for women, found no important differences, and presented their results for both sexes combined. Table 1 presents the main results of their study.

Table 1. Classification of risk factors for fracture related to bone mass loss(taken from reference [45])

High risk (15%)*	Moderate risk (18%)*	No risk (8%)*	Unclassifiable (59%)*
Aging (> 70–80 years)	Gender (female)	Consumption of caffeine	Alcohol intake
Low body weight[a]	Smoking (active)	Consumption of tea	Long-term immobilization
Weight loss[b]	Low sunlight exposure (low or none)	Menopause[j]	Type of menopause[k]
Physical inactivity[c]	Family history of osteoporotic fracture[d]	Nulliparity	Menopausal discomfort
Corticosteroids	Surgical menopause[e]	Consumption of fluoridated Water	Prior practice of athletics
Anticonvulsants	Early menopause (<45 years)[f]	Thiazide diuretics	High number of children
Primary hyperparathyroidism[†]	Short fertile period (<30 years)[g]		Old age at parity
Diabetes mellitus type I[†]	Late menarche (>15 years)[h]		Other reproductive factors[l]
Anorexia nervosa[†]	No lactation		Male hypogonadism
Gastrectomy[†]	Low calcium intake (<500–850 mg/day)[i]		Other hormonal factors in men
Pernicious anemia[†]	Hyperparathyroidism (N/S)		Mineral nutrient intake
Prior osteoporotic fracture	Hyperthyroidism		Dietary deficiency of vitamin D
	Diabetes mellitus (type II or N/S)		Dietary deficiency of vitamin C
	Rheumatoid arthritis		High-protein diet
			Deficient nutritional intake indicators
			Other dietary habits
			Prostaglandin inhibitors[m]
			Thyroid hormone replacement therapy
			Non-thiazide diuretics
			Tamoxifen
			Anti-ulcer agents
			Metabolism and gastrointestinal absorption disorders[n]
			Other thyroid disorders[o]
			Respiratory diseases[p]
			Neoplasm[q]
			Paget's disease
			Peptic ulcer
			Thalassemia
			Lithiasis

N/S, not specified.

*Percentage of total risk factors identified.

†There is little available scientific evidence for this risk factor, its quality also being moderate. However, the available studies show a consistent and significant increase in fracture risk.

[a]BMI (body mass index) lower than 20–25 kg/m2 or weight under about 40 kg.

[b]Greater than 10% (compared with the usual young or adult weight, or weight loss in recent years).

[c]No physical activities are performed regularly (walking, climbing stairs, carrying weights, housework, gardening, or other).

[d]Hip fracture in first-degree relatives was the most frequently studied risk factor.

[e]Due to bilateral oophorectomy.

[f]Before 45 years.

[g]Duration less than 30 years.

[h]From 15 years.

[i]Less than 500–850 mg/day (patient's age and gender should be assessed) or low/no consumption of dairy products such as milk (<1 glass/day) or cheese.

[j]Menopause, due to nonspecified cause or by oophorectomy (unspecified uni- or bilateral).

[k]Surgical vs natural.

[l]Includes those related to menstrual cycle, miscarriages, hysterectomy and tubal ligation.

[m]Includes aspirin and other nonsteroidal anti-inflammatories.

[n]Includes hepatic cirrhosis, chronic renal failure, regional enteritis, gastrointestinal resection.

[o]Includes goiter, adenoma and unspecified glandular disorders.

[p]Includes asthma, chronic bronchitis and emphysema.

[q]Includes endometrial carcinoma, breast carcinoma and any type of neoplasm.

We also identified a recent review (2005) that assessed risk factors for fractures.[46] While not a systematic review, the paper is authored by leaders in the World Health Organization osteoporosis community, and presents summaries of data originally presented in research articles (primarily by the co-authors). Included in this paper is a table summarizing their assessment of risk factors for osteoporotic fractures, with an additional notation indicating those factors that confer extra risk over and above that determined by BMD. That table is reproduced here as Table 2.

Table 2. Risks for osteoporotic fractures (taken from reference [46])

Female gender	Premature menopause
Age[a]	Primary or secondary amenorrhoea
	Primary and secondary hypogonadism in men
Asian or Caucasian race	Previous fragility fracture[a]
Low BMD	Glucocorticoid therapy[a]
High bone turnover[a]	Family history of hip fracture[a]
Poor visual acuity[a]	Low body weight[a]
Neuromuscular disorders[a]	Cigarette smoking[a]
	Excessive alcohol consumption[a]
	Prolonged immobilisation
	Low dietary calcium intake
	Vitamin D deficiency

[a]These characteristics capture aspects of fracture risk over and above that provided by BMD

Of the 176 articles that we identified which assessed risk factors for osteoporosis in men, we identified those that concentrated on factors for which prior reviews demonstrated an uncertain evidence base and factors that might have specific importance to the VA population.

These data were discussed with the Evidence Synthesis Project Steering Committee. After reviewing the risk factors about which there was still some uncertainty, they identified diabetes mellitus type II or NOS, spinal cord injury and alcohol use as factors most relevant to the VA and directed us to pursue a more detailed evaluation of articles relevant to these factors.

We therefore selected the 45 articles that measured one of these risk factors and assessed them with a brief screening form (Appendix A). Table 3 presents the results. There were 38 articles that assessed alcohol use, 15 that assessed diabetes mellitus and 4 that assessed spinal cord injury. Eight studies were cohorts, 9 were case control studies, and 28 were cross sectional in design. Almost all studies adjusted for, or in some way accounted for confounding by age, body weight, cigarette smoking, and physical activity, but adjustments for other potential risk factors were rare and variable.

Because of inherent problems with temporal ambiguity we rejected the cross sectional studies. Because of data supporting the superiority of cohort studies over case control studies,[47] we focused on the cohort studies. We identified seven articles assessing alcohol, but rejected one[48]

as data from this cohort were included in another study. Thus there were six articles about alcohol use. We identified one cohort assessing diabetes mellitus type II. We identified four relevant studies of osteoporosis in patients with spinal cord injury (SCI), one case control study and three cross-sectional studies.

Each study was assessed for quality using criteria suggested by Hayden & colleagues.[24] Tables 4a-c and Table 5 present descriptive details.

SYNTHESIS

Alcohol Use and Osteoporotic Fracture

Three articles assessed the relationship between alcohol intake and osteoporotic fractures.[49-51] Use of this outcome measure means that alcohol's effect on bone density and its known effect on predisposing to falls are both included in the association. It was not possible to pool studies as the articles measure the exposure variable, alcohol use, in different ways: self report of units per day, days per week, or weekly number and kind of drinks. The measurement of alcohol exposure is known to be very sensitive to how self-report questions are asked.[52] Study size was in general large, with 3,000-17,800 participants. On the Hayden items, these three studies scored modestly, with only 2 or 3 items being scored as fully satisfied, the remaining, being partly satisfied or unsure.

The two studies that assessed the association of units per day of alcohol intake and hip fracture both reported a statistically significant association. In the first of them, which also combined several other studies (in Canada, Australia, and the Netherlands) into a single analysis, assessed the relationship between self-reported alcohol use and hip fracture or osteoporotic fracture in about 6,000 men followed on average about 4 years.[49] Alcohol use was measured once at entry and fractures were assessed by self-report with medical record verification. In a multivariate analysis adjusted for age, body mass index, and smoking (but not physical activity), a statistically significant association was seen in alcohol intake exceeding 3 units per day (3 units/day, RR hip fracture=1.91; 4 units/day, RR hip fracture=2.84, RR any osteoporotic fracture=1.81).

The second study, three cohorts in Copenhagen that were originally assembled to assess cardiovascular disease were re-assessed for the incidence of hip fracture as determined by inpatient admission for same in a national database of hospital discharges.[51] More than 17,000 men were followed for 10 or more years. Alcohol intake was measured once, at entry into the study. In multivariate models adjusted for age, physical activity, body mass index, and other variables, a statistically significant association between baseline self-reported alcohol use and hip fracture was seen for categories of drinking exceeding 4 units per day (4-6 units/day, RR=1.75; 6-10 units/day, RR=1.84, >10 units/day, RR=5.28).

The third study to assess the relationship between alcohol intake and fracture came from the European Prospective Osteoporosis Study, which enrolled 3,173 men and followed them for about 4 years.[50] Alcohol use was measured once at entry and was reported as frequency in days per week. Vertebral fractures were assessed with baseline and follow-up spinal radiographs. In bivariate analyses, increasing alcohol intake had modest associations with vertebral fractures (RR approximately 1.2 to 1.6) but these were not statistically significant.

Alcohol Use and Bone Mineral Density

Three articles assessed the relationship between alcohol use and bone mineral density as measured by DXA.[53-55] Again, we could not pool these studies because they measured the use of alcohol in different ways. These studies were much smaller than the studies assessing fractures, with 150-507 persons being assessed. These studies scored somewhat better on the Hayden items, with 3, 4, and 5 items being scored as fully satisfied.

These three studies reached inconclusive results. A study of 278 from Framingham reported a statistically significant association between self-reported alcohol intake greater than seven ounces per week and decreased BMD only at the radial shaft. There were nonsignificant decreases in BMD at the trochanter and the lumbar spine.[55]

A study of the Rancho Bernardo cohort assessed 811 white men and reported a moderate positive effect of consuming alcohol three or more times per week on femoral neck BMD measured four years later. Non-significant positive associations were also reported for BMD measured at the spine and total hip.[54] The third study in this group assessed 308 men in Spain.[53] Participants completed a postal survey at entry and again at four years regarding health habits, including units per week of alcohol consumption. BMD was measured by DXA and performed at baseline and again at four years. No statistically significant association between alcohol intake and change in BMD was found.

Summary of Alcohol Use and Osteoporotic Fracture Evidence

Taken together, this group of studies suggests that alcohol intake is probably associated with an increase in hip fractures, but only at high rates of consumption. The lack of association reported in the European Prospective Osteoporotic study could be due to lack of specificity in the classification of alcohol consumption, as this study could not assess high rates of consumption. The available evidence fall short of proof because the strength of the association is modest (RR<2) and within the level where confounding is still a serious concern, and imprecision in the classification of alcohol consumption by self-report is present in all studies. With regard to BMD, these is no compelling evidence that alcohol intake is associated with lower BMD. (GRADE quality of evidence: Alcohol and Fractures = Low; Further research is very likely to have an important impact on our confidence in the estimate of effect and is likely to change the estimate; Alcohol and BMD = Very Low; any estimate of effect is very uncertain.)

Diabetes Mellitus Type II

We identified only one cohort study that assessed the association between Type II diabetes mellitus and osteoporosis.[56] This study assessed 998 older male participants in the Health ABC study, which was conducted in Pittsburgh and Memphis. The presence of diabetes was assessed by self-report and a fasting blood glucose (and follow-up two hour oral glucose tolerance test in selected participants). Bone density was determined using DXA at the proximal femur at entry and at follow-up. Duration of follow-up was four years. In multivariable models adjusting for age, baseline BMD, weight change, smoking status, renal status, and other variables, there was no association between the presence of diabetes and femoral neck or total hip BMD. On the Hayden criteria, this study scored very strongly, fully satisfying all six items.

Spinal Cord Injury

We identified four relevant studies of osteoporosis in patients with SCI, one case control study and three cross-sectional studies[43,57-59] (Table 5). A large body of literature was also identified that assessed changes in BMD over time in patients with SCI.

The case control study compared 17 New Zealander SCI male patients between the ages of 17 and 52 who were matched for age, height, weight and time spent in physical activity with able-bodied male controls (many of the participants were elite sportsmen)[57]. Eleven of the SCI patients were tetraplegic and six paraplegic. BMD by DXA was measured for the total body, arms, legs, left hip and lumbar spine. There were significant differences in mean T-scores of the legs and hip between the SCI and control groups; and, mean t-scores in the SCI patients were consistent with osteoporosis in the legs and trochanter and osteopenia in the femoral neck and Wards triangle.

Further supporting the association between SCI and bone loss were the three cross-sectional studies. The first evaluated 41 veteran SCI patients with a mean age of 55 for predictors of osteoporotic fractures in SCI patients[43]. This study found a high prevalence of osteoporosis (61%) and osteopenia (19.5%) in the patients studied as well as a high prevalence of previous fracture (34%). Controlling for age and duration of SCI, BMD was a strong predictor of fracture with the risk of fracture increasing 2.6 times for each unit decrease in BMD T-score. Another cross-sectional study evaluated the BMD of 46 male SCI patients with a mean age of 32 and compared this to age-matched reference values and found significantly lower BMD Z-scores in the proximal femur and distal forearm but not in the lumbar spine[58]. Patients with a history of at least two weeks of immobilization after spine surgery had significantly lower BMD Z-scores in the proximal femur but not in the lumbar spine or distal forearm. Patients with complete SCI had lower BMD Z-scores in the lumbar spine compared to patients with incomplete SCI.

The last cross-sectional study evaluated 41 Turkish SCI patients of which 32 were male with a mean age of 34.4 years[59]. BMD Z-scores were significantly higher in the upper extremities for paraplegic patients when compared to tetraplegic patients; and, when evaluating paraplegic patients alone, BMD Z-scores were significantly higher in the upper extremities than the lower extremities. This study also demonstrated that BMD Z-scores were significantly higher in SCI patients with incomplete injuries versus those with complete injuries, in those with spastic versus flaccid paralysis, and in those with a shorter duration of injury.

As mentioned above, there were a number of longitudinal studies which evaluated changes in BMD for patients with SCI. These studies did not meet our criteria for in-depth review but overall were consistent in demonstrating decreasing BMD over time in SCI patients. Four of these studies assessed veterans with SCI.[40-42,44] These studies support the hypothesis that SCI is a risk factor for osteoporosis.

Summary of Spinal Cord Injury and Osteoporosis or Osteoporotic Fracture
Taken together, these case-control and cross-sectional studies of SCI patients indicate that osteoporosis is significantly more likely in patients with SCI compared to non-SCI patients; that BMD worsens with duration of SCI ; and, that decreases in BMD are more significant in bones distal to the SCI level. Fracture risk also appears elevated but the evidence is less robust.

CONCLUSIONS

We found an older high quality meta analysis assessing numerous risk factors, and a limited number of articles specific to the risk factors alcohol use, diabetes mellitus type II and spinal cord injury. Based on these findings, our review suggests the following.

1. *Strong predictors of an increased risk of osteoporosis in men include age, low body weight, physical inactivity, and weight loss.* (GRADE quality of evidence = High; further research is very unlikely to change our confidence on the estimate of effect.)

2. *Certain health conditions and medications also are strong or moderate predictors of an increased risk of osteoporosis in men.* The most relevant to VA are prolonged systemic corticosteroid therapy and androgen deprivation (in the context of prostate cancer treatment). (GRADE quality of evidence = Moderate; further research is likely to have an important impact on our confidence in the estimate of effect and may change the estimate.)

3. *Alcohol use is probably associated with an increase in osteoporotic fractures, but is not clearly associated with an increase in osteoporosis as measured by BMD.* (GRADE quality of evidence: Fractures = Moderate; further research is likely to have an important impact on our confidence in the estimate of effect and may change the estimate; BMD = Very Low; any estimate of effect is very uncertain.)

4. *There is no evidence that diabetes mellitus type II is a significant risk factor for osteoporosis in men.* (GRADE quality of evidence: Low; further research is very likely to have an important impact on our confidence in the estimate of effect and is likely to change the estimate.)

5. *Spinal cord injury is associated with an increase risk of osteoporosis and possibly osteoporotic fractures.* (GRADE quality of evidence: BMD=Moderate; further research is likely to have an important impact on our confidence in the estimate of effect and may change the estimate; Fractures=Low; further research is very likely to have an important impact on our confidence in the estimate of effect and is likely to change the estimate.)

Table 3. Descriptive Data about Risk Factor Articles

Risk Factor Assessed:	Number of Articles
Alcohol... 38	
Diabetes Type II or NOS................................15 *includes 12 articles that also assessed alcohol	
Spinal Cord Injury.......................................4	

Study Design:	
Cohort..8	
Case-Control.....................................9	
Cross Sectional..................................28	

Outcomes Assessed:	
cDXA..28	
Site:	
Spine....................17	
Femur....................23	
Other....................9	
Osteoporotic Fracture...........................19	
Assessed by:	
X-ray....................11	
Medical Record Review........8	
Administrative data.........4	
Diary.....................4	
Other Bone Measurements.........................8	
Ultrasound.................2	
Other......................8	

Covariates Adjusted for:	Percent of Articles
Age..82%	
Low body weight.................................84%	
Weight loss.....................................9%	
Physical inactivity/prolonged immobilization.71%	
Corticosteroid use..............................36%	
Anticonvulsant use..............................16%	
Hyperparathyroidism.............................9%	
Diabetes Type I.................................0%	
Gastrectomy.....................................13%	
Hypogonadism, primary or secondary.............16%	
Poor visual acuity.............................2%	
Previous osteoporotic fracture.................29%	
Cigarette smoking..............................89%	
Vitamin D deficiency...........................16%	
Low dietary calcium intake.....................60%	
Family history of osteoporosis.................31%	
Hyperthyroidism................................20%	
Rheumatoid arthritis...........................18%	
High bone turnover rate........................4%	

Table 4a. Cohort Studies Assessing Alcohol as a Risk Factor, Outcome Measure: Fracture Occurrence

Article	Population	Enrolled /Included in analysis	Duration of follow up	Alcohol Consumption Definition	Fracture Occurrence assessed	Covariates adjusted for	Quality Measurement			Results
							Study Participation (SP) / Study Attrition (SA) / Prognostic Factor Measurement (PFM)	Outcome Measurement (OM) / Confounding Measurement (CM) / Analysis (A)		
Kanis, 2005[49]	3 cohort populations with mean ages 60, 70, 67 years	5939 / 5939	27,968 person yrs	Units / day	Diary Medical Record Review	Age Low body weight Smoking	SP: Partly SA: Unsure PFM: Yes	OM: Partly CM: Partly A: Yes		Alcohol intake of 3 units/day associated with increased RR of 1.91 for hip fracture. Alcohol intake of 4 units/day associated with increased RR of 1.81 for any osteoporotic fracture and increased RR of 2.84 for hip fracture.
Roy, 2003[50]	European men mean age 63.1 years	NR / 3173	3.8 years	5-6, 3-4, 1-2 days/wk	X-ray	Age Low body weight Inactivity Smoking Low calcium intake	SP: Partly SA: Unsure PFM: Yes	OM: Yes CM: Yes A: Partly		Alcohol intake was not associated with a significant increase in risk of vertebral fracture.
Holdrup, 1999[51]	Pooled data from 3 Danish cohorts mean age 50.5 years	17,868 / 17,868	13.6 years	Weekly number & kind of drinks	Administrative data Medical Record Review	Age Low body weight Inactivity Smoking	SP: Partly SA: Partly PFM: Yes	OM: Yes CM: Partly A: Yes		The relative risk of hip fracture was increased for men who drank 4 or more units per day (RR=1.75) and increased with increasing numbers of drinks/week (RR 5.28 for >10 units/day)

BMD=Bone Mass Density, NR=Not Reported, OP=Osteoporosis, RR =Relative Risk

Table 4b. Cohort Studies Assessing Alcohol as a Risk Factor, Outcome Measure: BMD

Article	Population	Enrolled /Included in analysis	Duration of follow up	Alcohol Consumption Definition	BMD		Refe-rence Stan-dard	Covariates adjusted for	Quality Measurement		Results
					Site	T-score			Study Participation (SP) / Study Attrition (SA) / Prognostic Factor Measurement (PFM)	Outcome Measurement (OM) / Confounding Measurement (CM) / Analysis (A)	
Naves, 2005[53]	Spanish men with mean age of 64 years	229 / 150	4 years	Units, unit= 10grams	Femur Spine	<-2.5=OP	Unclear	Age Low body weight Inactivity Smoking Low Calcium Intake Family History of OP fracture	SP: Yes SA: Yes PFM: Yes	OM: Partly CM: Yes A: Partly	Alcohol intake not significantly associated with change in BMD
Bakhireva 2004[54]	American men with mean age of 70.8 years	818 / 507	4 years	Drink >=3 days/wk v. <=2 days/wk	Femur Spine	<=-2=OP	Male	Age Low body weight Weight loss Inactivity Smoking Low calcium intake	SP: Yes SA: Partly PFM: Partly	OM: Yes CM: Yes A: Partly	Alcohol intake >=3 days/wk associated with decreased odds of bone loss at femoral neck (OR 0.68), but not at the spine
Hannan, 2000[55]	Elderly American men	NR / 278	4 years	Current vs. non user, grams/wk	Femur Spine	NR	NA	Age Low body weight Weight loss Inactivity Smoking Vitamin D deficiency Low calcium intake	SP: Yes SA: Partly PFM: Yes	OM: Yes CM: Yes A: Yes	Alcohol intake >= 7oz/wk associated with significant decrease in BMD at the radius, but not at the femoral neck or lumbar spine

BMD=Bone Mass Density, NR=Not Reported, NA=Not applicable, OP=Osteoporosis

Table 4c. Cohort Studies Assessing Diabetes Type II or NOS as a Risk Factor, Outcome Measure: BMD

Article	Population	Enrolled /Included in analysis	Duration of follow up	Presence of Diabetes Defined	BMD			Covariates adjusted for	Quality Measurement		Results
					Site	T-score	Refe-rence Stan-dard		Study Participation (SP) / Study Attrition (SA) / Prognostic Factor Measurement (PFM)	Outcome Measurement (OM) / Confounding Measurement (CM) / Analysis (A)	
Schwartz, 2005[56]	American men with mean age of 73.8 years	NR / 998	4 years	History Blood work (FBG) (75gOGTT)	Femur	NR	NA	Age, Inactivity Low body weight Weight Loss Corticosteroid use Smoking Low calcium intake	SP: Yes SA: Yes PFM: Yes	OM: Yes CM: Yes A: Yes	Diabetes type 2 not associated with significant change in BMD

BMD=Bone Mass Density, NR=Not Reported, NA=Not Applicable, OP=Osteoporosis, FBG=Fasting Blood Glucose, OGTT=Oral Glucose Tolerance Test

Table 5. Studies Assessing Spinal Cord Injury as a Risk Factor, Outcome Measure: BMD and/or Fracture Occurrence

Article	Population	Study Design	Cases /Controls Included OR Sample Size	Spinal Cord Injury Definition	Site	BMD T-score	Reference Standard	Fracture Occurrence Assessed	Covariates adjusted for	Quality Measurement Study Participation (SP) Study Attrition (SA) Prognostic Factor Measurement (PFM)	Quality Measurement Outcome Measurement (OM) Confounding Measurement (CM) Analysis (A)	Results
Jones, 2002[#108 3]	SCI patients in New Zealand, mean age 32 years	Case Control	17 cases 17 controls	Descriptive: Number of quadriplegic/para plegic; incomplete v. complete	Spine, Femur Radius, Finger Calcaneus Total body, arms, legs	<-2.5=OP	Young Adult Mean	Not assessed	Age Low body weight Inactivity	SP: Partly NA PFM: Partly	OM: Partly CM: No A: Yes	BMD values of total body, leg, and hip were significantly lower in SCI patients than in the controls
Lazo, 2001[#138 6]	Veteran SCI patients associated with the Hines VA, median age 55 years	Cross Sectional	45	American Spinal Injury Association Classification	Femur	NR	Male	X-ray Diary	Age	SP: Partly NA PFM: Yes	OM: Yes CM: No A: Yes	Controlling for age and SCI duration, each unit t-value decrement in BMD at the femoral neck increased the risk of fracture 2.8 times.
Sabo, 2001[#138 0]	Caucasian SCI patients <50 years living in Germany ; mean age 32	Cross Sectional	46	Frankel Score, Neuro Level Assessment	Spine, Femur, Radius	Z-score, NR	Age-related Reference	Not assessed		SP: No NA PFM: Yes	OM: Yes CM: No A: Partly	Compared with age-matched reference values, SCI patients had decreased BMD in the proximal femur and distal forearm. Post-operative immobilization and complete lesions were associated with lower BMD.
Demirel, 1998[#138 2]	SCI patients from the Istanbul Physical Medicine and Rehabilitation Centre; mean age 36	Cross Sectional	32	American Spinal Injury Association criteria for level of injury	Arms, Legs	Z-score, NR	Age-matched Z-score	Not assessed	Age Low body weight High bone turnover rate	SP: Partly NA PFM: Yes	OM: Partly CM: No A: Partly	BMD values were significantly higher in the upper extremities than in the lower extremities in paraplegic patients and BMD values in the upper extremities were significantly lower in quadriplegics compared to paraplegics.

SCI=Spinal Cord Injury, BMD=Bone Mass Density, NR=Not Reported, NA=Not applicable, OP=Osteoporosis

Key Question #2: Are there any validated tools (outside of DXA-determined central bone density) to screen for osteoporosis in men?

CONCEPTUAL FRAMEWORK

The clinical diagnosis of osteoporosis in men can be made in two ways: through the occurrence of a fragility fracture or based on bone density criteria. Fragility fractures typically occur after a prolonged decrease in bone density and quality and are the hallmark of osteoporotic bone disease. In 1994, the World Health Organization defined osteoporosis as a bone mineral density of greater than 2.5 standard deviations (T-score, -2.5) below that of a young healthy population. While this definition was originally proposed for postmenopausal women, it has also been used to define osteoporosis in men.

Use of the WHO-recommended threshold T-score of -2.5 has substantially simplified the clinical diagnosis of osteoporosis. Establishing a T-score threshold is useful and practical because substantial evidence suggests that each standard deviation decrement in bone density roughly doubles fracture risk. As such, bone density is an excellent tool for identifying those at high risk for future fracture. A simple causal pathway with bone density as the key determining factor for fracture risk (i.e., from normal bone density, to osteoporotic bone density, to fracture) is one way to conceptualize the progression of osteoporotic bone disease (Figure 2a). However, while bone density measurement is one of the best tools currently available to assess fracture risk, it is at best an imperfect predictor of future fracture.

Recent evidence, particularly from the National Osteoporosis Risk Assessment (NORA), which evaluated bone density and fracture history in over 200,000 postmenopausal women, reveals that the majority of osteoporotic fractures actually occur in those with a bone density T-score greater than -2.5. This is principally due to the poor sensitivity of central bone densitometry (reported to be around 70%) in identifying those who fracture. Although those without "osteoporosis" by T-score have lower rates of fracture than those with osteoporosis by T-score, there are much greater numbers of people with T-scores in the former category. These findings suggest that an alternate model of osteoporosis disease progression, one which incorporates multiple risk factors, is necessary to fully understand osteoporosis and identify those who will ultimately fracture (Figure 2b).

CONCEPTUAL FRAMEWORK FOR PROGRESSION OF OSTEOPOROSIS

Figure 2a. Bone Mineral Density-Centric Simple Model

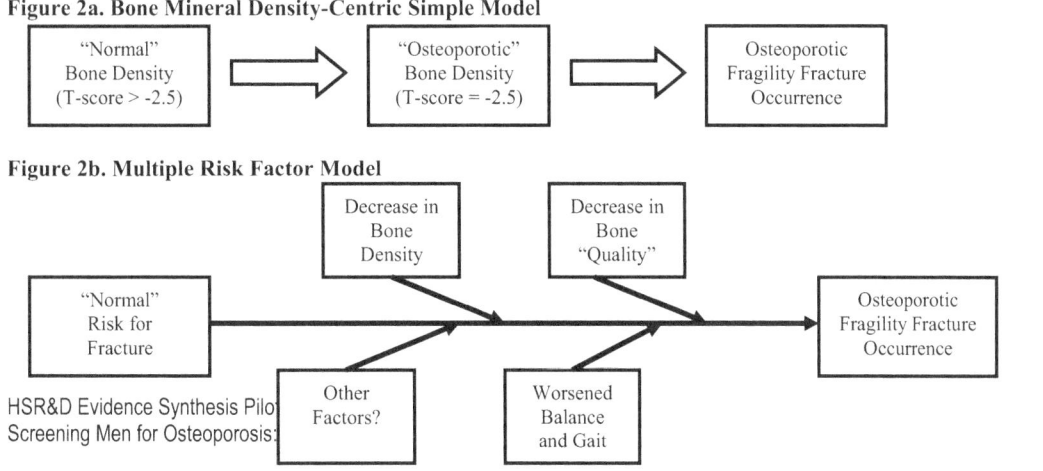

Figure 2b. Multiple Risk Factor Model

In this context, screening is defined as performing a test to identify the condition in persons who are asymptomatic. An evaluation of a screening test requires its comparison to a "gold standard" method for identifying the condition.

As there are two commonly used "gold standard" reference tests (i.e., bone mineral density and fracture occurrence) for the diagnosis of osteoporosis, studies evaluating osteoporosis screening tests can be broadly divided into two categories: 1) those that assess a test against a bone density measurement; and 2) those that assess a test against a fracture occurrence. As such, diagnostic studies that evaluate screening tests against both bone density and studies that evaluate screening tests against fracture occurrence are important for review and included in our analysis.

As bone mineral density is often employed as a "gold standard" reference test, we do not specifically examine the test characteristics of central bone density (DXA) as a screening modality in this section. A recent cost-effectiveness analysis was presented in abstract form, at the American Society of Bone and Mineral Research[60]. This study used microsimulation Markov modeling to assess a policy of universal DXA screening in men combined with five years of bisphosphonate therapy for those men found to have osteoporosis (using the young female reference standard). For patients without a prior non-spine fracture, estimated costs per year of quality-adjusted life year varied from $248,000 to $143,000 to $78,000 to $30,000 by the age at which screening was done (65, 70, 75 and 80 years of age, respectively.) This indicates that universal screening with DXA is unlikely to be cost-effective. An evaluation of DXA, and the values used to diagnose osteoporosis and the evidence regarding the relationship with osteoporotic fracture occurrence, is the topic of Key Question #3, found on page 37.

The published literature suggests that male osteoporosis is a significantly underdiagnosed condition. While osteoporosis screening tools, such as quantitative ultrasound, have been assessed in women, little research has been performed on validating such screening tools in men. We reviewed the literature to identify studies that evaluated a screening osteoporosis index test against a reference test (i.e., bone density or fracture occurrence) in men. Our goal was to assess the test performance characteristics of tests in men and determine the validity of these tests for screening in male osteoporosis.

DESCRIPTION OF EVIDENCE

Our search of *PubMed* identified 27 potentially relevant studies (See Figure 1, page 9). Descriptive information about these studies is displayed in Evidence Table 1 (see Appendix B). Of the 27 studies, 4 identified a veteran population. Twenty-one of the studies did not report the characteristics of the population; four had an Asian population; one had a Filipino population; one was other. The male sample size ranged from 33 to 6,860. In ten of the articles the population was unselected; eight included an elderly population; six used referrals; and three recruited patients from a specific clinic. Seven studies evaluated ultrasound (index test) against central dual x-ray absorptiometry (DXA, reference test); five studies evaluated osteoporosis screening questionnaires versus central DXA; and nine studies evaluated ultrasound versus fracture occurrence.

QUALITY EVALUATION

Quality as assessed using the QUADAS instrument showed that almost all of the articles scored adequately on description of the selection criteria, the ability of the reference test to correctly classify the condition, the time period between the index test and the reference test, the sample receiving the reference test, the independence of the reference test, the description of the index test and the reference test, the generalizability to clinical practice, the reporting of uninterruptible test results. Conversely, almost no report indicated that interpretation of either the reference test or the index test was performed without knowledge (or "blind") to the other test results. In 13 of 27 (48%), the representativeness of the enrolled population to a VA population was not clear. In almost half of studies (12 of 27), withdrawals from the study were either not explained or unclear, and in only half of studies (14 of 27) were patients selected representative of a population that might be eligible for screening in the VA. Thus, in this application, the QUADAS instrument had limited ability to distinguish between studies based on quality.

In terms of total score, none of the studies met all of the QUADAS criteria. However, 24 out of the 27 articles (88%) scored positive on at least 60% or more of the criteria. In studies of the efficacy of treatments, validation studies of the criteria of Jadad and of the Delphi list both found empirical evidence that a threshold of 60% of the criteria being met distinguished better quality studies from lesser quality studies.[61,62] Until such time as empirical studies with QUADAS are available, it seems reasonable to use the 60% threshold for classifying studies with QUADAS. Hence, most of the studies we evaluated were of good quality.

SCREENING TEST GROUPINGS

We found substantial heterogeneity in the original authors' use of thresholds both for the index test and reference test. Additionally, several studies did not provide key information, such as sample size by group. We reviewed available data and used clinical judgment to group studies into categories of comparisons for further quantitative analysis (Tables 6a-c). Using **central DXA as the reference standard**, we analyzed studies evaluating: ultrasound versus central DXA; and questionnaires versus central DXA. Using **fracture occurrence as the reference standard**, we reviewed studies evaluating ultrasound versus fracture occurrence. We did not pool data for other index and reference test combinations because of the heterogeneous nature of the data.

Table 6a. Study Test: Ultrasound vs. Reference Test: cDXA detailed comparison

STUDIES INCLUDED IN ANALYSIS

Article	Population	Study Test: Ultrasound				Reference Test: cDXA			Sens	Spec	Variance		Data Pooling	
		Machine	Location	Measurement	Units	Machine	Location	Units			Sens	Spec	Osteoporosis	Threshold
Gudmunds-dottir, 2005[20]	Unselected	Lunar Achilles+	Calcaneus L	SI	T Score	Hologic QDR 4500	LS, FN, TH	T Score	X	X			Total hip DXA T-score <-2.5 vs >-2.5	<0(risk) vs >=0(non-risk) <-0.5(risk) vs >=-0.5(non-risk) <-1.0(risk) vs >=-1.0(non-risk)
													Femoral neck BMD T-score <=-2.5 vs >-2.5	<0(risk) vs >=0(non-risk) <-0.5(risk) vs >=-0.5(non-risk) <-1.0(risk) vs >=-1.0(non-risk)
													Central DXA T-score <-1.5 vs >=-1.5	<0(risk) vs >=0(non-risk)
Kung, 2005[63]	Elderly	Hologic Sahara	Calcaneus R	QUI (SI?)	T Score	Hologic QDR 2000+	LS, F	T Score	X	X	X	X	Femoral Neck BMD T-score <=-2.5 vs >-2.5	<=-1.2(risk) vs >-1.2(low risk)
Adler, 2003a[19]	Referral	Hologic Sahara	Calcaneus	QUI (SI?)	T Score	Hologic QDR 4500	LS, FN, TH	T Score	X	X	X	X	T-score <=-2.0 vs >-2.0	<=-1.5(risk) vs >-1.5(non-risk)
Mulleman, 2002[64]	Referral	Lunar Achilles	Calcaneus	BUA, SOS & SI	T Score	Hologic QDR 2000	LS, PF	T Score	X		X		BMD (FN, LS, TH) <-2.5 vs >=-2.5	<-2.5(risk) vs >=-2.5 (non-risk)
													SI T-score <-2.5 vs >=-2.5	<-2.5(risk) vs >=-2.5 (non-risk)
													BMD (FN, LS, TH) <-1.0 vs >=-1.0	<-1.0 (risk) vs >=-1.0(non-risk)
													SI T-score <-1.0 vs >=-1.0	<-1.0 (risk) vs >=-1.0(non-risk)
Adler, 2001[27]	Referral	Hologic Sahara	Calcaneus	QUI (SI?)	T Score	Hologic 1000-W	LS, FN, TH	T Score	X	X	X	X	Central DXA T-score <-1.5 vs >=-1.5	<0(risk) vs >=0(non-risk) <-0.5(risk) vs >=-0.5(non-risk) <-1.0(risk) vs >=-1.0(non-risk) <-1.5(risk) vs >=-1.5(non-risk) <-2.0(risk) vs >=-2.0(non-risk) <-2.5(risk) vs >=-2.5(non-risk)
													Central DXA T-score <-2.0 vs >=-2.0	<0(risk) vs >=0(non-risk) <-0.5(risk) vs >=-0.5(non-risk) <-1.0(risk) vs >=-1.0(non-risk) <-1.5(risk) vs >=-1.5(non-risk) <-2.0(risk) vs >=-2.0(non-risk) <-2.5(risk) vs >=-2.5(non-risk)
													Central DXA T-score <-2.5 vs >=-2.5	<0(risk) vs >=0(non-risk) <-0.5(risk) vs >=-0.5(non-risk) <-1.0(risk) vs >=-1.0(non-risk) <-1.5(risk) vs >=-1.5(non-risk) <-2.0(risk) vs >=-2.0(non-risk) <-2.5(risk) vs >=-2.5(non-risk)

STUDIES NOT INCLUDED IN ANALYSIS (no data on sensitivity/specificity)

Article	Population	Machine	Location	Measurement	Units	Machine	Location	Units
Lynn, 2005[65]	Elderly	Hologic Sahara	Calcaneus R	QUI (SI?)	Unit-less	Hologic QDR 4500 W	LS, PF	T Score
Grampp, 2001[66]	Unselected	Lunar Achilles	Calcaneus	SI	T Score	Hologic QDR 4500	LS, FN	T Score
Montagnani, 2001[67]	NR	DBM Sonic	Phalanx	UBPI, QUS	Unit-less	Hologic QDR 4500	LS, FN, TH	T Score

Sens=Sensitivity, Spec=Specificity, LS=Lumbar Spine, FN=Femoral Neck, TH=Total Hip, PF=Proximal Femur, SI=Stiffness Index, BUA=Broad-band ultrasound attenuation, SOS=Speed of sound, BMD=Bone Mass Density, UBPI=Ultrasound Bone Profile Index, US=Quantitative Ultrasound

Table 6b. Study Test: Questionnaire vs. Reference Test: cDXA detailed comparison

STUDIES INCLUDED IN ANALYSIS

Article	Population	Study Test: Questionnaire			Reference Test: cDXA			Sens	Spec	Variance		Data Pooling	
		Name	Key Inputs	Units	Machine	Location	Units			Sens	Spec	Threshold	
Kung, 2005[63]	Elderly	Clin Risk Assess Tool	Age, Weight	Score -11-10	Hologic QDR 2000 +	LS, F	T Score	X	X			Femoral neck BMD T-score <=-2.5 vs >-2.5	<=-1(risk) vs >-1 (low risk)
Li-Yu, 2005[15]	Referral	Osteoporosis Screening Tool for Asians (OSTA)	Age, Weight	Lo, Med, Hi Risk	GE Lunar DPX-IQ	FN	T Score	X	X	X	X	BMD T-score <=-2.5 vs >-2.5	<=-1 (high/medium risk) vs >-1 (low risk)
Lynn, 2005[65]	Elderly	Male Osteoporosis Screening Tool (MOST)	Weight, QUI*	Score 0 - 8	Hologic QDR 4500 W	LS, PF	T Score	X	X			Lumbar spine, total hip or Femoral neck BMD T-score <-2.5 vs >-2.5	>3(risk) vs <3(non-risk)
Adler, 2003b[35]	Referral	Osteoporosis Screening Tool (OST)	Age, Weight	Cutoff 3,2,1	Hologic QDR 4500	LS, FN, TH	T Score	X	X	X	X	DXA T-score <=-2.5 vs >-2.5	<4(high/moderate risk) vs >=4(low risk) <=-2(high risk) vs >-2 (moderate/low risk)

STUDIES NOT INCLUDED IN ANALYSIS (no data on sensitivity/specificity)

Article	Population	Name	Key Inputs	Units	Machine	Location	Units
Adler, 2003a[19]	Referral	Questionnaire	Weight, Heel BMD, steroids, race	Score 0 - 14	Hologic QDR 4500	LS, FN, TH	T Score

Sens=Sensitivity, Spec=Specificity, LS=Lumbar Spine, FN=Femoral Neck, TH=Total Hip, PF=Proximal Femur, BMD=Bone Mass Density

Table 6c. Study Test: Ultrasound vs. Reference Test: Fracture Occurrence detailed comparison

| Article | Population | Machine | Study Test: Ultrasound | | | Reference Test: Fracture Occurrence |
			Location	Measurement	Units	Location & Details
Gonnelli, 2005[68]	Referral	Lunar Achilles +	Calcaneus	SI	percent	Fragility Fractures: vertebral, wrist, pelvis, femur
Varenna, 2005[69]	Other	Lunar Achilles	Calcaneus	SI, BUA, SOS	unitless, db/Mhz, m/s	Low energy fractures since age 50
Rothenberg, 2004[70]	Other	Hologic Sahara	Calcaneus	Estimated BMD	gm/cm2, T score	Self reported fractures, followed up by phone call
Welch, 2004[71]	Other	McCue CUBA	Calcaneus	BUA	db/MHz	Self reported vertebral, hip, wrist fractures or diagnosis of osteoporosis
Mulleman, 2002[64]	Referral	Lunar Achilles	Calcaneus nondom	SI	T Score	Vertebral, other; low trauma; vertebral fractures: X-ray with > 15% decrease in vertebral height
Donaldson, 1999[72]	Elderly	Walker Sonix 1001	Calcaneus	BUA	db/MHz	Any since 50, By recall; minimum trauma
Stewart, 1995[73]	Other	Walker Sonix UBA 575	Calcaneus	BUA	db/MHz	Patients with vertebral fractures vs controls
Travers-Gustafson. 1995[74]	Elderly	Osteo-Technology Signet	Patella	AVU	m/sec	Fractures since age 40, experts assessed fracture reports, low trauma
Bauer2004[75]	Elderly	Hologic Sahara	Calcaneus	BUA	db/MHz	Hip and non-spine fractures in older men

Sens=Sensitivity, Spec=Specificity, LS=Lumbar Spine, FN=Femoral Neck, TH=Total Hip, PF=Proximal Femur, BMD=Bone Mass Density

CENTRAL DXA AS REFERENCE TEST

Ultimately, we were able to pool only studies evaluating calcaneal ultrasound versus central DXA and those evaluating Osteoporosis Self-Assessment Tool (OST) versus central DXA (Table 6a-b). There were studies comparing ultrasound to cDXA that we could not include in our pooled analysis because they lacked data to calculate the sensitivity and specificity.[65-67] Details of these analyses are presented below and in graphical format, along with a pooled ROC curve from a recently published meta-analysis of the utility of calcaneal ultrasound versus central DXA in women,[76] in the following series of figures (Figures 3a-d, 4, 5).

Calcaneal Ultrasound versus Central DXA

Calcaneal ultrasound, in which an ultrasound probe is placed on either heel, has the advantages of being portable, inexpensive, and radiation-free. Ultrasound measurements are often reported as T-scores (standardized units) of the quantitative ultrasound index (QUI). However, there is no commonly accepted threshold for a positive QUI reading, and our review showed that thresholds from 0 to -2.5 have been used.

Given this heterogeneity in thresholds, we were able to incorporate data from only 3 studies for our summary sensitivity and specificity measurements.[19,27,63] We found that using a calcaneal ultrasound T-score of -1.0, calcaneal ultrasound had a sensitivity of 75% and a specificity of 66% to diagnose bone density-determined osteoporosis (central DXA T-score of < -2.5) (Figure 3a). When the calcaneal ultrasound threshold was decreased to -1.5, specificity improved to 78% but sensitivity dropped to 47%. We were able to construct a ROC curve from one study evaluating male veterans[27] (Figure 3b), which varied calcaneal ultrasound thresholds from -1.5 to -2.5. Superimposing these ROC curves onto a recently reported ROC curve of calcaneal ultrasound in primarily women (Figure 3c) showed these curves to be similar, suggesting that calcaneal ultrasound likely performs comparably in men as in women (Figure 3d).

The Osteoporosis Self-Assessment Tool (OST) versus Central DXA

The Osteoporosis Self-Assessment Tool, which uses a subject's age and weight to develop a risk score (equation: [(weight in kilograms – age in years) x 0.2], truncated to an integer), is a simple test which has been primarily evaluated and validated in women. More recently, a number of evaluations have been performed in men, with particular attention to the veteran population.[35] Similarly to calcaneal ultrasound, there is no commonly accepted OST risk score threshold. Our review showed that thresholds from -1 to 3 have been used (Table 6b).

Pooling data from two studies of evaluations of Asian men (Chinese and Filipino), we found that at an OST risk score of -1, the OST had a sensitivity of 81% and specificity of 68% to diagnose bone density-determined osteoporosis. In the only study of OST in Veterans (Figure 4), the authors found that at an OST threshold of 3, the OST had a sensitivity of 93% and specificity of 66%. Sensitivity decreased to 75% and specificity increased to 80% when the OST threshold was decreased to 1. Of note, at all thresholds evaluated, the OST had higher sensitivity and specificity than calcaneal ultrasound, although this analysis is limited by the paucity of data points available and therefore no definitive conclusions can be drawn.

Summary Figure 5 graphs all results from all articles with relevant data, and the meta-analytic result for the ROC curve in primarily women[76] (data in red). The figure shows that all studies assessing ultrasound reported results that are close to the pooled ROC curve for primarily women. The studies assessing OST reported results above the pooled ROC curve, suggesting OST may be more accurate than ultrasound.

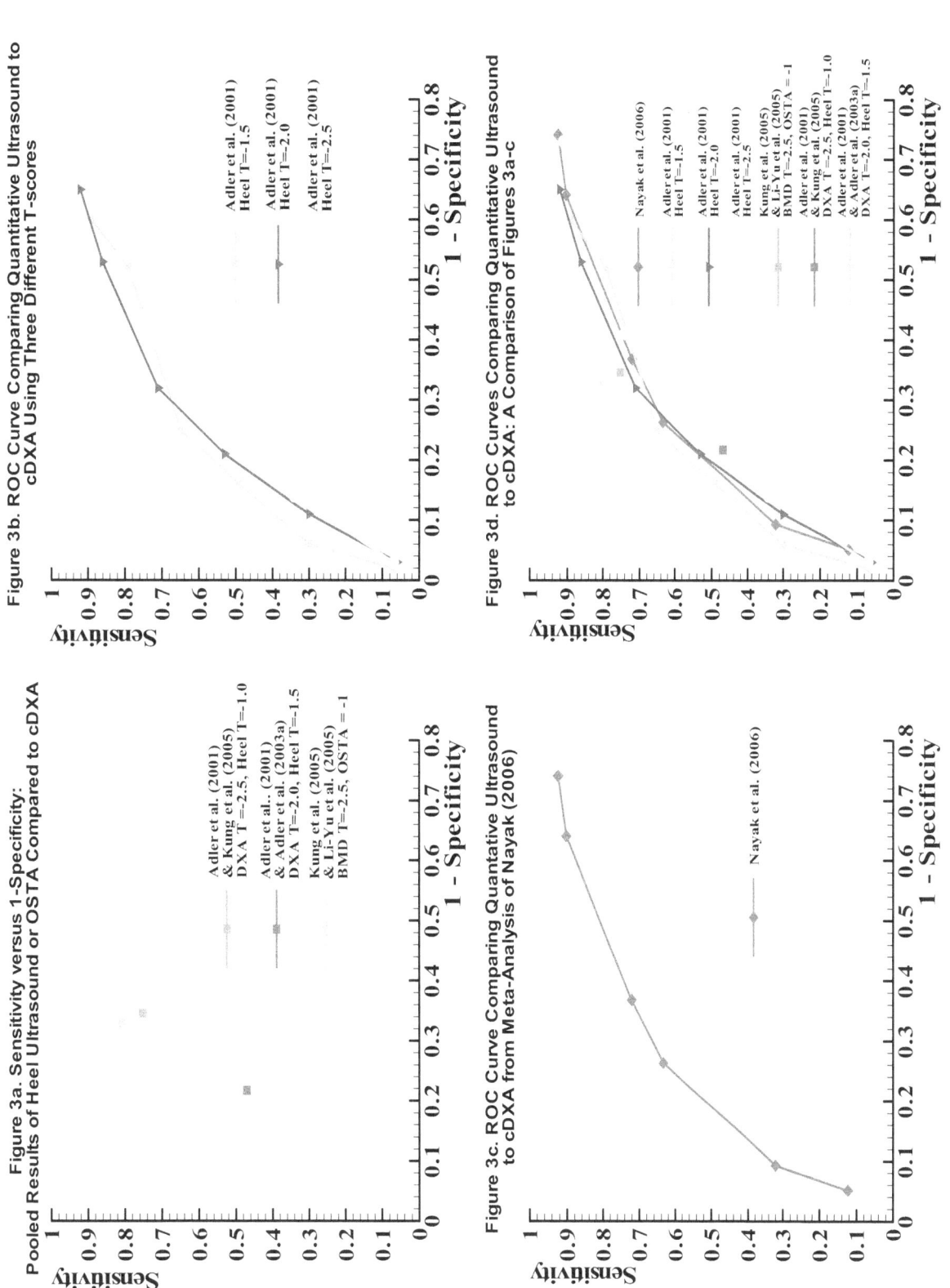

Figure 3a. Sensitivity versus 1-Specificity: Pooled Results of Heel Ultrasound or OSTA Compared to cDXA

Figure 3b. ROC Curve Comparing Quantitative Ultrasound to cDXA Using Three Different T-scores

Figure 3c. ROC Curve Comparing Quantative Ultrasound to cDXA from Meta-Analysis of Nayak (2006)

Figure 3d. ROC Curves Comparing Quantitative Ultrasound to cDXA: A Comparison of Figures 3a-c

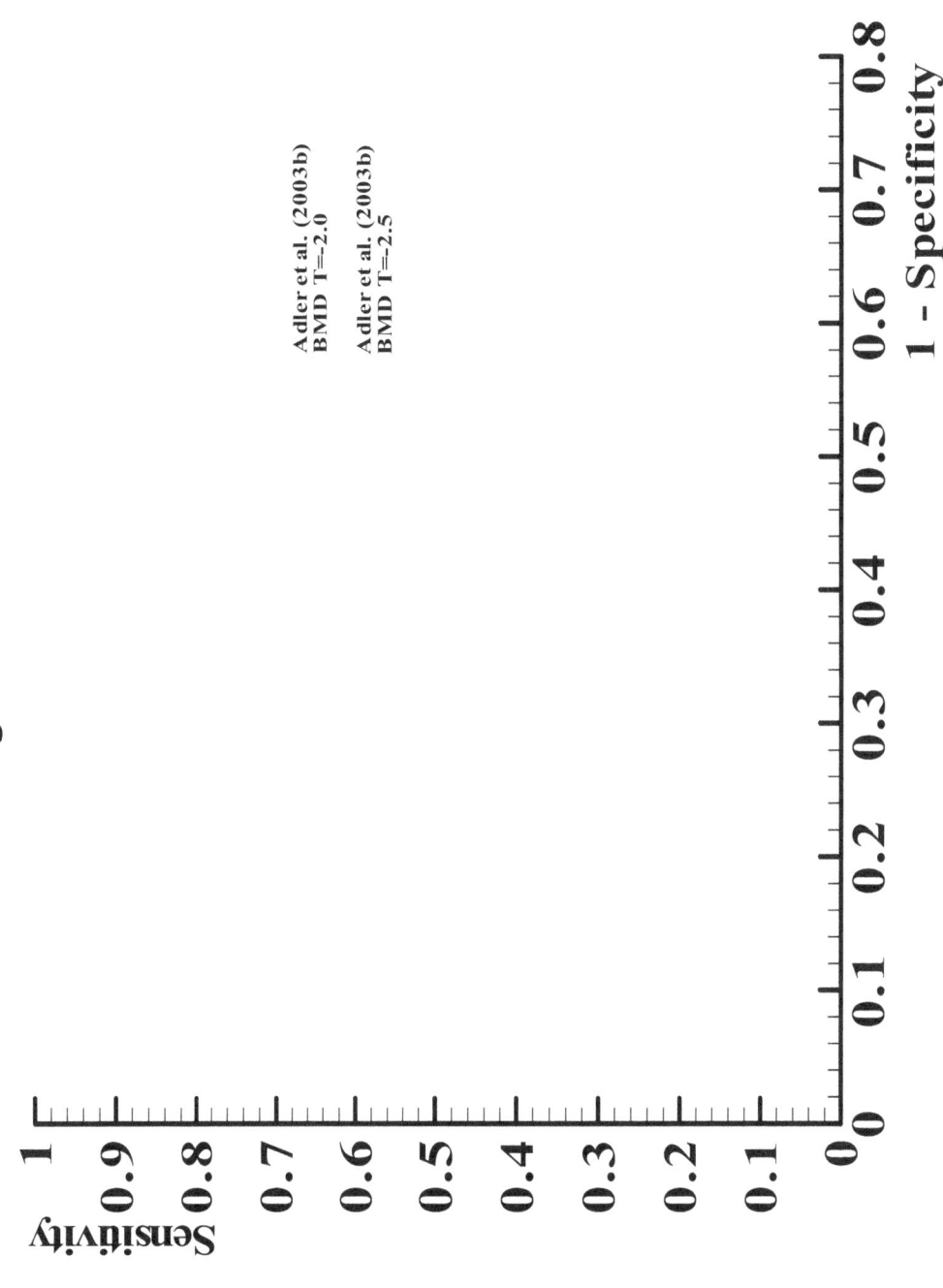

Figure 4. ROC Curve Comparing OST to cDXA using Two Different T-Scores

Adler et al. (2003b)
BMD T=-2.0

Adler et al. (2003b)
BMD T=-2.5

Figure 5. ROC Curves and Individual Study Sensitivity versus 1-Specificity (All Studies)

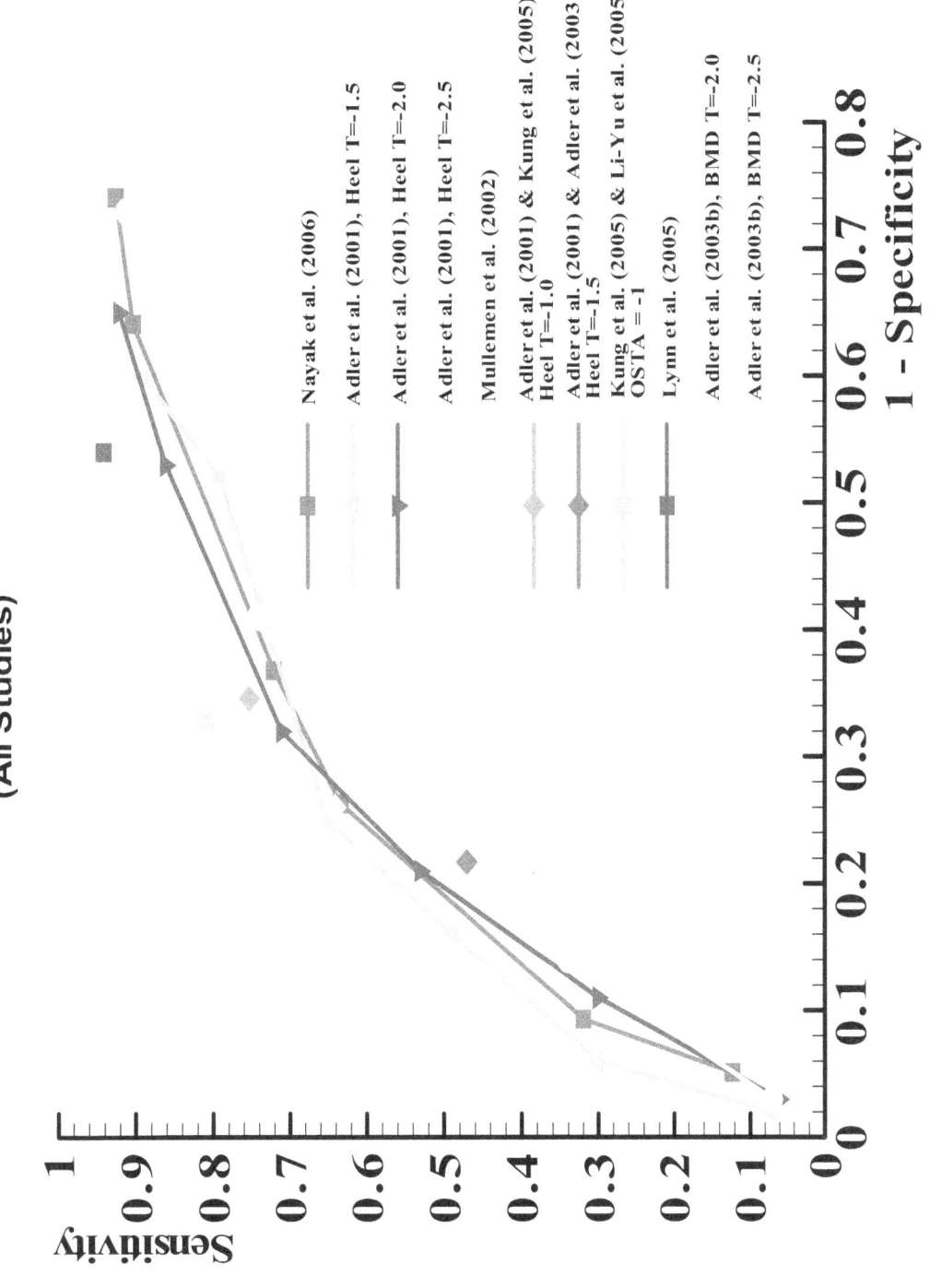

Legend:
- Nayak et al. (2006)
- Adler et al. (2001), Heel T=-1.5
- Adler et al. (2001), Heel T=-2.0
- Adler et al. (2001), Heel T=-2.5
- Mullemen et al. (2002)
- Adler et al. (2001) & Kung et al. (2005) Heel T=-1.0
- Adler et al. (2001) & Adler et al. (2003a) Heel T=-1.5
- Kung et al. (2005) & Li-Yu et al. (2005) OSTA = -1
- Lynn et al. (2005)
- Adler et al. (2003b), BMD T=-2.0
- Adler et al. (2003b), BMD T=-2.5

FRACTURE OCCURRENCE AS REFERENCE TEST

Eighteen studies used fractures occurrence as the reference test, with: ten evaluating ultrasound as the index test; two evaluating quantitative CT, and one each evaluating peripheral bone density, central bone density, x-ray, bone structural parameters, linear photon absorptiometry, and a multivariate scoring model (Table 6c). However, we could not pool data from these studies given the heterogeneity of the data although we provide a qualitative assessment of studies evaluating ultrasound against fracture occurrence below. We narratively summarized the nine studies that assessed ultrasound to occurrence of fragility fractures.[64,68-75]

Calcaneal Ultrasound versus Fracture Occurrence

Calcaneal ultrasound appears to be independently associated with and moderately predictive of fragility fracture in men. One study found that each standard deviation reduction in ultrasound measurement resulted in an approximate two-fold increase in hip fractures that was independent of age and other clinical variables and comparable to findings in elderly women.[69] Similarly, an abstract published from the ongoing and pivotal MrOS Study, a population-based study of older men, found that each SD reduction in calcaneal ultrasound measurement was associated with an increased risk of hip (relative hazard, 2.0, 1.3-3.5) and non-spine fracture (relative hazard, 1.7, 1.4-2.0).[75] Finally, another study found that ultrasound stiffness parameters had a strong association (odds ratio 3.2, 2.3-4.5) with prior fragility fracture.[68]

More controversial is whether the combination of bone density measurements and calcaneal ultrasound to assess for fractures is better than either test alone. One study found that both bone mineral density of the hip (odds ratio, 3.4) and ultrasound (odds ratio, 3.2) were strongly associated with fragility fracture.[68] If bone density and ultrasound results were combined, the odds ratio for fracture association increased to 6.1. However, an analysis of ROC curves for hip fracture prediction from the MrOS study for: ultrasound alone (AUC, 0.84); bone mineral density alone (AUC, 0.85); and the combination of the two (AUC 0.85) suggested that the combining ultrasound and bone mineral density was not superior to using either modality alone.[75] As such, it remains unclear as to whether an optimal male osteoporosis screening program should include bone density, ultrasound, or a combination of these two or other test modalities.

CONCLUSIONS

Although the limited number of studies published on male osteoporosis screening tools precludes drawing definitive conclusions on these tests, our review suggests the following:

1) *There is no evidence to suggest that calcaneal ultrasound performs differently in men than in women.* Our pooled data points and the ROC curve we constructed to evaluate calcaneal ultrasound against a reference standard of bone density appeared comparable to a

recently published ROC curve on calcaneal ultrasound that included studies primarily evaluating women. In addition, we found evidence that calcaneal ultrasound measurements were predictive of or associated with fractures in men at similar levels as those published for women. As such, we find no evidence indicating that calcaneal ultrasound should perform any differently in men as it does in women. The available data fall short of proof, but suggest that calcaneal ultrasound performs comparably in men as in women. (GRADE quality of evidence = Moderate; further research is likely to have an important impact on our confidence in the estimate of effect and may change the estimate.)

2) *The OST appears to have comparable (and possibly better) test characteristics than calcaneal ultrasound in diagnosing DXA-determined osteoporosis.* The OST, a questionnaire which incorporates only age and weight, appears to perform as well or better than ultrasound in predicting DXA-determined osteoporosis. Supporting this conclusion, one of the studies identified assessed Veterans, and found test characteristics similar to our pooled analysis. This simple tool appears promising and could potentially be easily incorporated into a mass osteoporosis screening program. However, caution must be exercised as two of the three studies we quantitatively analyzed enrolled exclusively men from Asia. In addition, all of these studies evaluated the OST against DXA, and not against fracture occurrence, which is the critical outcome of interest. Our results suggest that more evaluation of this test is urgently warranted and necessary. (GRADE quality of evidence = Low; further research is very likely to have an important impact on our confidence in the estimate of effect and is likely to change the estimate.)

3) *Although calcaneal ultrasound does not appear to be a particularly good test at diagnosing DXA-determined osteoporosis, it is a strong, independent predictor of fractures in men.* Although ultrasound may not perform exceptionally well at predicting a particular bone mineral density score, it appears to perform well in identifying a population of patients who will fracture, the endpoint that clinicians and patients ultimately care about. Both bone density and ultrasound can identify populations who will fracture, although these populations do not appear to fully overlap. Ultrasound may be identifying deficits in other bone parameters, such as bone quality, which may not be identified through bone density measurement. However, as almost all clinical trials of osteoporosis drugs recruited patients based on a bone density score and not an ultrasound score, it remains to be determined if those identified at risk for fracture by ultrasound will benefit from our current osteoporosis drug armamentarium. This finding is likely to be true for all patients identified to be "at risk" through the screening modalities (e.g., osteoporosis screening questionnaires) evaluated in this review, as it is not clear that current pharmacologic interventions decrease fracture risk in such populations given the lack of clinical trial evaluation in these specific groups. (GRADE quality of evidence = Moderate; further research is likely to have an important impact on our confidence in the estimate of effect and may change the estimate.)

4) *Limited data are available on other screening modalities and there is a large gap in our understanding of osteoporosis screening tests in men.* Our comprehensive review identified only 26 studies in total evaluating osteoporosis screening tests in men. We were only able to perform limited quantitative analyses on two screening tests: calcaneal ultrasound and the OST. It remains unclear if other screening tests, such as quantitative CT, other types of

questionnaires, or peripheral bone density measurements, might also be useful as screening tests in men. As such, there is a large, and currently unmet, need for additional research in this field of study.

5) *A majority of the studies compared a screening test against DXA and not fracture occurrence*. Most of the studies we identified evaluated a screening test against the gold standard of central DXA rather than fracture occurrence. The relevant clinical outcome is fracture occurrence, and studies assessing their relationship are needed. In order to interpret the clinical utility of such studies, though, evidence is needed about the effectiveness of therapies to prevent fracture occurrence in men identified as high risk based on calcaneal ultrasound, or OST, etc.

Key Question 3: What values of BMD determined by DXA (and by different DXA techniques) have been used to diagnose osteopenia and osteoporosis; and what is the evidence regarding the relationship between differing definitions and the development of osteoporotic fractures?

Our review identified 31 articles evaluating the association between BMD as measured by DXA and the risk of fractures in men. Most of these articles indicated that BMD is a strong predictor of fracture risk in men and femoral neck BMD is a stronger predictor than lumbar spine BMD. Almost all studies assessed BMD as a standardized measure (in terms of T-score or Z-score) and not in terms of grams of bone mineral content per centimeter squared.

Risk of fracture per standard deviation decrease in BMD varied by study. One large meta-analysis of 12 cohort studies[77] found that the gradient of risk for an osteoporotic fracture per standard deviation decrease in z-score in men ("gradient of risk" = RR/SD) was 1.6 and the gradient of risk for a hip fracture per standard deviation decrease in z-score in men was 2.42. Another large prospective cohort study[78] found a 3.2 time increased risk of hip fracture per sex-specific SD decrease in total hip BMD.

Virtually all studies evaluating the relationship between BMD and osteoporosis in men defined osteoporosis as a BMD more than 2.5 standard deviations below the mean for young adults ("T-score"). However, whether to use a young female or a young male reference range when evaluating BMD in men is an area of controversy that is not possible to resolve with existing data. In a summary statement from the International Conference on Osteoporosis in Men in 2002, international experts "agreed to disagree" on this issue, each marshalling data to support their own position.

In an article from this conference, a summary of the evidence favoring use of the female reference range was presented. Proponents of this cite studies that have demonstrated that measurement of BMD at the hip expressed as a T-score using the female reference standard predicts fracture risk similarly in men and women. By far the largest study identified was a meta-analysis of 12 cohort studies that collectively included 9891 men, 29082 women and 168,366 person years.[77] The "gradient of risk" (RR/SD) for each SD decrease in BMD using sex and age-specific standard deviations (Z-scores) was virtually identical in men and women; and, was not significantly different from the "gradient of risk" using the standard deviation of a young female reference range (T-scores). For instance, in men the gradient of risk for osteoporotic fractures was 1.6 using a sex and age-specific reference range and was 1.55 using a young female reference range. In women, the gradient of risk for osteoporotic fractures was 1.53 using a sex and age-specific reference range and 1.56 using a young female reference range. Currently, this is the primary evidence behind the argument that the reference range used in men and women should be the same, and should be the female range. The study shows not only that gradient of risk is the same but also that the absolute risk is the same in men and women using the female range.

Additionally, some studies have demonstrated that men and women at the same age with the same absolute BMD at the hip have an equal likelihood of hip fracture.[79] Thus, these experts argue that osteoporosis in men should be defined as it is in women, using T-scores derived from a young healthy female reference population.

Critics of this conclusion, raise several concerns. First, they argue that, despite the large numbers of patients included in this pooled analysis, the data are imprecise because different populations are mixed together. Important heterogeneity in effect may be obscured. Second, these critics point to a large prospective study demonstrating a much stronger relationship in men than in women between hip BMD & subsequent fracture[78] as evidence that there are important gender differences to be discovered and dealt with. Furthermore, they point out that using a young female reference range underestimates the expected prevalence of osteoporosis in men. In one study by Melton[80] evaluating the association of BMD with hip fracture risk, the prevalence of osteoporosis in men using a young healthy male reference range was 19.4% versus only 3.4% using a young healthy female reference range. In another study by Falkner,[81] prevalence estimates for osteoporosis in men differed depending on which reference range was utilized. This study also raised the question as to whether using the standard definition of osteoporosis (more than 2.5 standard deviations below the mean) is appropriate in men since the T-scores that best corresponded to the lifetime risk for osteoporotic fracture in men were significantly different from -2.5 (-1.9 using young male reference ranges and -1.5 using young female reference ranges). Thus, there is evidence that using female-specific reference ranges may significantly under detect osteoporosis in men and result in fewer men being identified who may, in fact, be at risk for osteoporotic fracture and might benefit from treatment.

Proponents of the female standard respond to these arguments by highlighting the fact that there are few data relating use of the male reference range and the 5- or 10-year risk of fracture.

Whether to utilize gender-specific reference ranges to determine T-scores when screening for osteoporosis remains an area of uncertainty and awaits further prospective studies evaluating the association of fracture and BMD. But a principle of screening is that it should be performed only when there is an effective health care strategy for early treatment.[82] Therefore, when deciding which reference range to choose given current limited information, it is helpful to evaluate how subjects were identified as candidates for osteoporosis therapies in randomized controlled trials that have demonstrated a benefit in reducing risk of osteoporotic fractures. In other words, a screening program to identify Veterans with osteoporosis would be rooted in current evidence when it identifies persons who are most similar to the subjects enrolled in the RCTs that we rely on to guide treatment. Table 7 presents information from all of the RCTs identified in an ongoing systematic review of therapies for osteoporosis (Comparative Effectiveness Review of Pharmacologic Therapies for Low Bone Density, Southern California Evidence Based Practice Center Draft Report) that reported data specific to men, using as outcome either fractures or any of several intermediate outcomes. Many of these studies used the existing presence of osteoporotic fractures as an entry criterion, and in that case the concept of "screening" does not apply. But in those studies that used BMD as measured by DXA as the entry criterion for low bone density, all used T-scores using the young male reference standard. Therefore, this is evidence that men identified with low bone density/osteoporosis using the young male reference standard (which is a larger percentage of the potentially osteoporotic population than would be identified using the young female standard, as discussed previously) will benefit from treatment. This does not account for the potential for heterogeneity in treatment effects.[27,66] In some RCTs, it has been shown that studies reporting a benefit in the enrolled population actually provided large benefit to only a portion of that population – usually the most severely affected – while providing no benefit or actually harming other enrolled patients, although the net "overall" result was still positive. Whether there is heterogeneity in treatment effects in the RCTs of treatment for men with low bone density is not known. However, until more definitive evidence is available, we believe it is most logically consistent for VA to identify men who might benefit from treatment for osteoporosis by adhering to the same conditions as were used in RCTs of osteoporosis treatment; namely, the young male reference standard. (GRADE quality of evidence = Low; further research is very likely to have an important impact on our confidence in the estimate of effect and is likely to change the estimate.)

Table 7. Entry Criteria of Trials Reporting Efficacy of Osteoporosis Treatment in Men.

Studies that Use Fracture Reduction as Outcome

Study	DXA Site	T-score	Reference	Includes Fragility Fracture	Treatment Assessed
Ringe 2006[83]	Lumbar Spine	<=-2.5	male	with or without	risedronate
Kaufman, 2005[84]	Femoral Neck	<=-2.0	male	with or without	risedronate
	Lumbar Spine or Proximal Femur	<=-2.0	male	no	teriparatide
Ringe, 2004[85] & Ringe, 2001[86]	Lumbar Spine	<-2.5	male	no	alendronate
Orwoll, 2003[54]	Proximal Femur or Lumbar Spine	<-2.0	male	no	teriparatide
	Femoral neck and Lumbar Spine	<=-2.0 FM & <=-1.0 LS	male	no	alendronate
Orwoll, 2000[87]	Femoral neck	<=-1.0	male	no	alendronate

Studies that Use Other Outcomes

Study	DXA Site	T-score	Reference	Includes Fragility Fracture	Treatment Assessed	Outcome
Shimon, 2005[88]	Lumbar Spine or Femoral Neck	<=-2.0	male	not inclusion criteria but reported in Table1	alendronate	BMD lumbar spine & femoral neck
Kurland, 2000[89]	Lumbar Spine or Femoral Neck	<=-2.5	male	not inclusion criteria but reported	parathyroid hormone	BMD lumbar spine & femoral neck
Toth, 2005[57]	Lumbar Spine or Femoral Neck	<-2.5	gender specific	no	intranasal salmon calcitonin therapy	BMD lumbar spine & femoral neck
	Femoral Neck and Lumbar Spine	<-2.0 FM & <-1.0 LS	male	no	alendronate	BMD lumbar spine & total spine
Drake, 2003[90]	Femoral Neck	<-1.0	male	yes	alendronate	
Laroche, 1998[91]	Lumbar Spine	<-2.5	male	lumbar spine BMD and/or fractures	fluoride, etidronate, calcitron	BMD
Trovas, 2002[92]	Lumbar Spine or Femoral Neck	<-2.5	male	no	nasal spray salmon calcitonin	BMD spine & femoral neck
Gonnelli, 2003[93]	Lumbar Spine or Femoral Neck	<=-2.5	male	not inclusion criteria, but reported	alendronate	BMD lumbar spine, femoral neck, total hip

40

BMD=Bone mass density

SUMMARY AND DISCUSSION

In this chapter, we describe the limitations of our review and meta-analysis and then present our conclusions. We also discuss the implications of our findings for future research.

Limitations

PUBLICATION BIAS

Our literature search procedures were extensive and included canvassing experts from academia regarding studies we may have missed. It was not possible to conduct formal tests for publication bias, but even with such tests it is not possible to exclude the possibility that such bias exists. Therefore, readers are cautioned about this possibility.

STUDY QUALITY

An important limitation common to systematic reviews is the quality of the original studies. Recent attempts to define elements of study design and execution that are related to bias have shown that in many cases, such efforts are not reproducible and do not distinguish study results based on bias. Therefore, the current approach is to avoid rejecting studies or using quality criteria to adjust the meta-analysis results. We did use the QUADAS criteria and those suggested by Hayden and colleagues as a descriptive measure of quality. As there is a lack of empirical evidence regarding study characteristics and their relationship to bias, we did not attempt to use other criteria. Other aspects of the design and execution of a trial may be related to bias, but we do not yet have good measures of these elements. Because of the small number of studies found, it was not possible to do sensitivity analyses based on study quality.

HETEROGENEITY

In our meta-analysis, it was not possible to calculate a test of heterogeneity. Clearly, the populations being assessed were different, and there were also important differences in how some key variables were measured, which diagnostic tests were used, and which reference standard for classifying osteoporosis was used, among others. This heterogeneity further limits our ability to draw strong conclusions.

APPLICABILITY OF FINDINGS

Green & Glasgow[94] provide a framework for evaluating the relevance, generalization, and applicability of research. Their framework includes assessing the participation rate, the intended target population, the representativeness of the setting, the representativeness of the individuals, and evaluating information about implementation and assessment of outcomes. As these data are rarely reported in the studies we reviewed, conclusions about applicability are necessarily weak.

Conclusions

With the above limitations in mind, we reached the conclusions displayed below.

KEY QUESTION #1: What are the prevalence of and risk factors for osteopenia, osteoporosis and osteoporotic fractures among men in general and among male Veterans specifically?

Prevalence

- There are no VA specific data on prevalence of osteopenia and osteoporosis in men.

- Applying NHANES III estimates of prevalence to veteran-specific enrollee data we estimate the prevalence of osteoporosis in male veterans of 200,000 – 400,000; and of osteopenia in male veterans of 2-3 million.

Risk Factors

- We found a high quality meta analysis, and a limited number of articles specific to the risk factors alcohol use, diabetes mellitus type II and spinal cord injury. Based on these findings, our review suggests the following.

- Strong predictors of an increased risk of osteoporosis in men include age, low body weight, physical inactivity, and weight loss. (GRADE quality of evidence = High; further research is very unlikely to change our confidence on the estimate of effect.)

- Certain health conditions and medications also are strong or moderate predictors of an increased risk of osteoporosis in men. The most relevant to VA are prolonged systemic corticosteroid therapy and androgen deprivation (in the context of prostate cancer treatment). (GRADE quality of evidence = Moderate; further research is likely to have an important impact on our confidence in the estimate of effect and may change the estimate.)

- Alcohol use is probably associated with an increase in osteoporotic fractures, but is not clearly associated with an increase in osteoporosis as measured by BMD. (GRADE quality of evidence: Fractures = Moderate; further research is likely to have an important impact on our confidence in the estimate of effect and may change the estimate; BMD = Very Low; any estimate of effect is very uncertain.)

- There is no evidence that diabetes mellitus type II is a significant risk factor for osteoporosis in men. (GRADE quality of evidence: Low; further research is very likely to have an important impact on our confidence in the estimate of effect and is likely to change the estimate.)

- Spinal cord injury is associated with an increase risk of osteoporosis and possibly osteoporotic fractures. (GRADE quality of evidence: BMD= Moderate; further research is likely to have an important impact on our confidence in the estimate of effect and may change the estimate; BMD = Very Low; any estimate of effect is very uncertain; Fractures=

Low; further research is very likely to have an important impact on our confidence in the estimate of effect and is likely to change the estimate.)

KEY QUESTION #2: Are there any validated tools to screen for osteoporosis in men?

- The evidence for screening tools for men is much more limited than for women. We were only able to synthesize evidence on two screening tools: calcaneal ultrasound and the Osteoporosis Screening Tool (OST).

- There is no evidence to suggest that calcaneal ultrasound performs differently in men than in women. (GRADE quality of evidence = Moderate; further research is likely to have an important impact on our confidence in the estimate of effect and may change the estimate.)

- The OST appears to have comparable (and possibly better) test characteristics than calcaneal ultrasound in diagnosing DXA-determined osteoporosis. (GRADE quality of evidence = Low; further research is very likely to have an important impact on our confidence in the estimate of effect and is likely to change the estimate.)

- Although calcaneal ultrasound does not appear to be a particularly good test at diagnosing DXA-determined osteoporosis, it is a strong, independent predictor of fractures in men. (GRADE quality of evidence = Moderate; further research is likely to have an important impact on our confidence in the estimate of effect and may change the estimate.)

- Limited data are available on other screening modalities and there is a large gap in our understanding of osteoporosis screening tests in men.

KEY QUESTION #3: What values of BMD determined by DXA (and by different DXA techniques) have been used to diagnose osteopenia and osteoporosis; and what is the evidence regarding the relationship between differing definitions and the development of osteoporotic fractures?

- The values of BMD determined by DXA that have been used are based on standard deviations (T-score) away from a reference standard, either young female or young male.

- Whether to use a young female or a young male reference range in order to identify men as "at risk" for osteoporotic fractures is an area of controversy that is not possible to resolve with existing data.

- Until more definitive evidence is available, we believe it is most logically consistent for VA to identify men who might benefit from treatment for osteoporosis by adhering to the same conditions as were used in the RCTs of osteoporosis treatment; namely, the young male reference standard. (GRADE quality of evidence = Low; further research is very likely to have an important impact on our confidence in the estimate of effect and is likely to change the estimate.)

FUTURE RESEARCH

Our review suggests that additional and extensive research is urgently needed to better understand the risk factors, prevalence, and application of screening tests for male osteoporosis. While osteoporosis has been extensively evaluated in women, comparably little work has been done in men. As the largest integrated health care system in the U.S., serving a population that is more than 95% male and 80% over the age of 50, these issues are of particular concern and importance to the VA.

In particular, we have identified three areas of future research in male osteoporosis that we believe to be of critical importance to the VA:

1. Determine the scope of the problem within the veteran population. We did not find any veteran-specific data on the prevalence of osteoporosis or osteopenia in male veterans. Applying our own calculations based on NHANES III data, we estimate up to 400,000 veterans may have osteoporosis and 3 million may have osteopenia. However, as the NHANES cohort was a relatively healthy sample of the U.S. population, and as Veterans tend on average to have more comorbidity than non-Veterans, our calculations may underestimate the prevalence of osteoporotic disease in Veterans. Research that attempts to quantify the number of the Veterans at risk for osteoporotic disease, such as those that evaluate a representative veteran population, will help the VA better understand the burden of current and future osteoporotic disease. Cross-sectional studies of association will be helpful to better define which Veterans are most likely to have osteoporosis.

2. Further elucidate the test characteristics of promising screening tests. Based on limited evidence, we find the OST to be a promising screening test that could potentially be widely employed for male osteoporosis screening. An advantage to the OST is that is can be easily applied with existing data and could require minimal effort to program a CPRS clinical reminder using age and weight, which could trigger a patient specific request for a DXA scan. However, only three studies that evaluated the OST, of which only one in our analysis assessed a Veteran population. Additional research effort should be focused on testing the sensitivity, specificity, and positive predictive value of the OST in Veterans.

3. Determine the optimal screening regimen for male osteoporosis in Veterans. Ultimately, the goal of a male osteoporosis screening program will be to determine and implement a sensitive yet cost-effective screening strategy. Future clinical research efforts should focus on evaluating and comparing different screening strategies. In addition, computer modeling, including cost-effectiveness analysis, should be used to aid decision-making on optimal resource allocation. Avaliable evidence suggests that universal screening with cDXA based on age is unlikely to be cost-effective: strategies of targeted screening with cDXA based on other risk factors have not been evaluated.

REFERENCES

1. Morris CA, Cabral D, Cheng H, Katz JN, Finkelstein JS, Avorn J, et al. Patterns of bone mineral density testing: current guidelines, testing rates, and interventions. J Gen Intern Med 2004; 19:783-90.

2. Pacini S, Aterini S, Ruggiero M, Gulisano M. Bone mineral density and anthropometric measures in normal and osteoporotic men. Ital J Anat Embryol 1999; 104:195-200.

3. Halling A, Persson GR, Berglund J, Johansson O, Renvert S. Comparison between the Klemetti index and heel DXA BMD measurements in the diagnosis of reduced skeletal bone mineral density in the elderly. Osteoporos Int 2005; 16:999-1003.

4. Stehman-Breen CO, Sherrard D, Walker A, Sadler R, Alem A, Lindberg J. Racial differences in bone mineral density and bone loss among end-stage renal disease patients. Am J Kidney Dis 1999; 33:941-6.

5. Oefelein MG, Resnick MI. The impact of osteoporosis in men treated for prostate cancer. Urol Clin North Am 2004; 31:313-9.

6. Bano G, Rodin DA, Pazianas M, Nussey SS. Reduced bone mineral density after surgical treatment for obesity. Int J Obes Relat Metab Disord 1999; 23:361-5.

7. Nguyen TV, Eisman JA, Kelly PJ, Sambrook PN. Risk factors for osteoporotic fractures in elderly men. Am J Epidemiol 1996; 144:255-63.

8. Maugeri D, Panebianco P, Barbagallo P, Malaguarnera M, Curasi MP, Russo MS, et al. Estrogens and euosteogenesis in men. Eur Rev Med Pharmacol Sci 1998; 2:189-92.

9. Wong PK, Spencer DG, McElduff P, Manolios N, Larcos G, Howe GB. Secondary screening for osteoporosis in patients admitted with minimal-trauma fracture to a major teaching hospital. Intern Med J 2003; 33:505-10.

10. Bass E, Campbell RR, Werner DC, Nelson A, Bulat T. Inpatient mortality of hip fracture patients in the Veterans Health Administration. Rehabil Nurs 2004; 29:215-20.

11. Looker AC, Orwoll ES, Johnston CC Jr, Lindsay RL, Wahner HW, Dunn WL, et al. Prevalence of low femoral bone density in older U.S. adults from NHANES III. J Bone Miner Res 1997; 12:1761-8.

12. Papaioannou A, Parkinson W, Ferko N, Probyn L, Ioannidis G, Jurriaans E, et al. Prevalence of vertebral fractures among patients with chronic obstructive pulmonary disease in Canada. Osteoporos Int 2003; 14:913-7.

13. Jorgensen HL, Hassager C. Improved reproducibility of broadband ultrasound attenuation of the os calcis by using a specific region of interest. Bone 1997; 21:109-12.

14. Karlsson KM, Sernbo I, Obrant KJ, Redlund-Johnell I, Johnell O. Femoral neck geometry and radiographic signs of osteoporosis as predictors of hip fracture. Bone 1996; 18:327-30.

15. Li-Yu JT, Llamado LJ, Torralba TP. Validation of OSTA among Filipinos. Osteoporos Int 2005; 16:1789-93.

16. Fink HA, Kuskowski MA, Orwoll ES, Cauley JA, Ensrud KE. Association between Parkinson's disease and low bone density and falls in older men: the osteoporotic fractures in men study. J Am Geriatr Soc 2005; 53:1559-64.

17. Kaptoge S, Armbrecht G, Felsenberg D, Lunt M, O'Neill TW, Silman AJ, et al. When should the doctor order a spine X-ray? Identifying vertebral fractures for osteoporosis care: results from the European Prospective Osteoporosis Study (EPOS). J Bone Miner Res 2004; 19:1982-93.

18. Yang NP, Lin T, Wang CS, Chou P. Community-based survey of low quantitative ultrasound values of calcaneus in Taiwan. J Clin Densitom 2003; 6:131-41.

19. Adler RA, Funkhouser HL, Petkov VI, Elmore BL, Via PS, McMurtry CT, et al. Osteoporosis in pulmonary clinic patients: does point-of-care screening predict central dual-energy X-ray absorptiometry? Chest 2003; 123:2012-8.

20. Gudmundsdottir SL, Indridason OS, Franzson L, Sigurdsson G. Age-related decline in bone mass measured by dual-energy X-ray absorptiometry and quantitative ultrasound in a population-based sample of both sexes: identification of useful ultrasound thresholds for osteoporosis screening. J Clin Densitom 2005; 8:80-6.

21. Hummer M, Malik P, Gasser RW, Hofer A, Kemmler G, Moncayo Naveda RC, et al. Osteoporosis in patients with schizophrenia. Am J Psychiatry 2005; 162:162-7.

22. Thomason K, West J, Logan RF, Coupland C, Holmes GK. Fracture experience of patients with coeliac disease: a population based survey. Gut 2003; 52:518-22.

23. Karadag F, Cildag O, Yurekli Y, Gurgey O. Should COPD patients be routinely evaluated for bone mineral density? J Bone Miner Metab 2003; 21:242-6.

24. Berntsen GK, Tollan A, Magnus JH, Sogaard AJ, Ringberg T, Fonnebo V. The Tromso Study: artifacts in forearm bone densitometry--prevalence and effect. Osteoporos Int 1999; 10:425-32.

25. Bessant R, Keat A. How should clinicians manage osteoporosis in ankylosing spondylitis? J Rheumatol 2002; 29:1511-9.

26. Xu SZ, Zhou W, Mao XD, Xu J, Xu LP, Ren JY. Reference data and predictive diagnostic models for calcaneus bone mineral density measured with single-energy X-ray absorptiometry in 7428 Chinese. Osteoporos Int 2001; 12:755-62.

27. Adler RA, Funkhouser HL, Holt CM. Utility of heel ultrasound bone density in men. J

Clin Densitom 2001; 4:225-30.

28. Colon-Emeric C, Yballe L, Sloane R, Pieper CF, Lyles KW. Expert physician recommendations and current practice patterns for evaluating and treating men with osteoporotic hip fracture. J Am Geriatr Soc 2000; 48:1261-3.

29. Iqbal F, Michaelson J, Thaler L, Rubin J, Roman J, Nanes MS. Declining bone mass in men with chronic pulmonary disease: contribution of glucocorticoid treatment, body mass index, and gonadal function. Chest 1999; 116:1616-24.

30. Yaturu S, DjeDjos S, Alferos G, Deprisco C. Bone mineral density changes on androgen deprivation therapy for prostate cancer and response to antiresorptive therapy. Prostate Cancer Prostatic Dis 2006; 9:35-8.

31. Conde FA, Sarna L, Oka RK, Vredevoe DL, Rettig MB, Aronson WJ. Age, body mass index, and serum prostate-specific antigen correlate with bone loss in men with prostate cancer not receiving androgen deprivation therapy. Urology 2004; 64:335-40.

32. Elliott ME, Drinka PJ, Krause P, Binkley NC, Mahoney JE. Osteoporosis assessment strategies for male nursing home residents. Maturitas 2004; 48:225-33.

33. Yeh SS, Phanumas D, Hafner A, Schuster MW. Risk factors for osteoporosis in a subgroup of elderly men in a Veterans Administration nursing home. J Investig Med 2002; 50:452-7.

34. Stanley HL, Schmitt BP, Poses RM, Deiss WP. Does hypogonadism contribute to the occurrence of a minimal trauma hip fracture in elderly men? J Am Geriatr Soc 1991; 39:766-71.

35. Adler RA, Tran MT, Petkov VI. Performance of the Osteoporosis Self-assessment Screening Tool for osteoporosis in American men. Mayo Clin Proc 2003; 78:723-7.

36. Townsend MF, Sanders WH, Northway RO, Graham SD Jr. Bone fractures associated with luteinizing hormone-releasing hormone agonists used in the treatment of prostate carcinoma. Cancer 1997; 79:545-50.

37. Villareal MS, Klaustermeyer WB, Hahn TJ, Gordon EH. Osteoporosis in steroid-dependent asthma. Ann Allergy Asthma Immunol 1996; 76:369-72.

38. Ohldin A, Floyd J. Unrecognized risks among Veterans with hip fractures: opportunities for improvements. J South Orthop Assoc 2003; 12:18-22.

39. Lazo MG, Shirazi P, Sam M, Giobbie-Hurder A, Blacconiere MJ, Muppidi M. Osteoporosis and risk of fracture in men with spinal cord injury. Spinal Cord 2001; 39:208-14.

40. Szollar SM, Martin EM, Sartoris DJ, Parthemore JG, Deftos LJ. Bone mineral density

and indexes of bone metabolism in spinal cord injury. Am J Phys Med Rehabil 1998; 77:28-35.

41. Szollar SM, Martin EM, Parthemore JG, Sartoris DJ, Deftos LJ. Densitometric patterns of spinal cord injury associated bone loss. Spinal Cord 1997; 35:374-82.

42. Szollar SM, Martin EM, Parthemore JG, Sartoris DJ, Deftos LJ. Demineralization in tetraplegic and paraplegic man over time. Spinal Cord 1997; 35:223-8.

43. Lazo MG, Shirazi P, Sam M, Giobbie-Hurder A, Blacconiere MJ, Muppidi M. Osteoporosis and risk of fracture in men with spinal cord injury. Spinal Cord 2001; 39:208-14.

44. Comarr AE, Hutchinson RH, Bors E. Extremity Fractures of Patients with Spinal Cord Injuries. American Journal of Surgery 1962; 103:732-9.

45. Espallargues M, Sampietro-Colom L, Estrada MD, Sola M, del Rio L, Setoain J, et al. Identifying bone-mass-related risk factors for fracture to guide bone densitometry measurements: a systematic review of the literature. Osteoporos Int 2001; 12:811-22.

46. Szulc P, Marchand F, Duboeuf F, Delmas PD. Cross-sectional assessment of age-related bone loss in men: the MINOS study. Bone 2000; 26:123-9.

47. Tovey FI, Godfrey JE, Lewin MR. A gastrectomy population: 25-30 years on. Postgrad Med J 1990; 66:450-6.

48. Nguyen TV, Center JR, Sambrook PN, Eisman JA. Risk factors for proximal humerus, forearm, and wrist fractures in elderly men and women: the Dubbo Osteoporosis Epidemiology Study. Am J Epidemiol 2001; 153:587-95.

49. Kanis JA, Johansson H, Johnell O, Oden A, De Laet C, Eisman JA, et al. Alcohol intake as a risk factor for fracture. Osteoporos Int 2005; 16:737-42.

50. Roy DK, O'Neill TW, Finn JD, Lunt M, Silman AJ, Felsenberg D, et al. Determinants of incident vertebral fracture in men and women: results from the European Prospective Osteoporosis Study (EPOS). Osteoporos Int 2003; 14:19-26.

51. Hoidrup S, Gronbaek M, Gottschau A, Lauritzen JB, Schroll M. Alcohol intake, beverage preference, and risk of hip fracture in men and women. Copenhagen Centre for Prospective Population Studies. Am J Epidemiol 1999; 149:993-1001.

52. Holmes-Walker DJ, Woo H, Gurney H, Do VT, Chipps DR. Maintaining bone health in patients with prostate cancer. Med J Aust 2006; 184:176-9.

53. Naves M, Diaz-Lopez JB, Gomez C, Rodriguez-Rebollar A, Serrano-Arias M, Cannata-Andia JB. Prevalence of osteoporosis in men and determinants of changes in bone mass in a non-selected Spanish population. Osteoporos Int 2005; 16:603-9.

54. Bakhireva LN, Barrett-Connor E, Kritz-Silverstein D, Morton DJ. Modifiable predictors of bone loss in older men: a prospective study. Am J Prev Med 2004; 26:436-42.

55. Hannan MT, Felson DT, Dawson-Hughes B, Tucker KL, Cupples LA, Wilson PW, et al. Risk factors for longitudinal bone loss in elderly men and women: the Framingham Osteoporosis Study. J Bone Miner Res 2000; 15:710-20.

56. Schwartz AV, Sellmeyer DE, Strotmeyer ES, Tylavsky FA, Feingold KR, Resnick HE, et al. Diabetes and bone loss at the hip in older black and white adults. J Bone Miner Res 2005; 20:596-603.

57. Jones LM, Legge M, Goulding A. Intensive exercise may preserve bone mass of the upper limbs in spinal cord injured males but does not retard demineralisation of the lower body. Spinal Cord 2002; 40:230-5.

58. Sabo D, Blaich S, Wenz W, Hohmann M, Loew M, Gerner HJ. Osteoporosis in patients with paralysis after spinal cord injury. A cross sectional study in 46 male patients with dual-energy X-ray absorptiometry. Arch Orthop Trauma Surg 2001; 121:75-8.

59. Demirel G, Yilmaz H, Paker N, Onel S. Osteoporosis after spinal cord injury. Spinal Cord 1998; 36:822-5.

60. Schousboe JT, Taylor BC, Fink HA, Bauer DC, Nyman JA, Kane RL, et al. Cost-Effectiveness of universal bone densitometry followed by treatment of those with femoral neck T-score <-2.5 compared to no densitometry or treatment in elderly caucasian men with or without prior fracture. American Society of Bone and Mineral Research 28th Annual Meeting 2006; Abstract.

61. Fauchet M, Andrieux P, Roux C, Sebert JL. Broadband ultrasound attenuation at the calcaneus measured using a new contact ultrasound unit. Rev Rhum Engl Ed 1998; 65:257-66.

62. Robinson RJ, Carr I, Iqbal SJ, al-Azzawi F, Abrams K, Mayberry JF. Screening for osteoporosis in Crohn's disease. A detailed evaluation of calcaneal ultrasound. Eur J Gastroenterol Hepatol 1998; 10:137-40.

63. Kung AW, Ho AY, Ross PD, Reginster JY. Development of a clinical assessment tool in identifying Asian men with low bone mineral density and comparison of its usefulness to quantitative bone ultrasound. Osteoporos Int 2005; 16:849-55.

64. Mulleman D, Legroux-Gerot I, Duquesnoy B, Marchandise X, Delcambre B, Cortet B. Quantitative ultrasound of bone in male osteoporosis. Osteoporos Int 2002; 13:388-93.

65. Lynn HS, Lau EM, Wong SY, Hong AW. An osteoporosis screening tool for Chinese men. Osteoporos Int 2005; 16:829-34.

66. Grampp S, Henk C, Lu Y, Krestan C, Resch H, Kainberger F, et al. Quantitative US of

the calcaneus: cutoff levels for the distinction of healthy and osteoporotic individuals. Radiology 2001; 220:400-5.

67. Montagnani A, Gonnelli S, Cepollaro C, Mangeri M, Monaco R, Gennari L, et al. Usefulness of bone quantitative ultrasound in management of osteoporosis in men. J Clin Densitom 2001; 4:231-7.

68. Gonnelli S, Cepollaro C, Gennari L, Montagnani A, Caffarelli C, Merlotti D, et al. Quantitative ultrasound and dual-energy X-ray absorptiometry in the prediction of fragility fracture in men. Osteoporos Int 2005; 16:963-8.

69. Varenna M, Sinigaglia L, Adami S, Giannini S, Isaia G, Maggi S, et al. Association of quantitative heel ultrasound with history of osteoporotic fractures in elderly men: the ESOPO study. Osteoporos Int 2005; 16:1749-54.

70. Rothenberg RJ, Boyd JL, Holcomb JP. Quantitative ultrasound of the calcaneus as a screening tool to detect osteoporosis: different reference ranges for caucasian women, african american women, and caucasian men. J Clin Densitom 2004; 7:101-10.

71. Welch A, Camus J, Dalzell N, Oakes S, Reeve J, Khaw KT. Broadband ultrasound attenuation (BUA) of the heel bone and its correlates in men and women in the EPIC-Norfolk cohort: a cross-sectional population-based study. Osteoporos Int 2004; 15:217-25.

72. Donaldson MM, McGrother CW, Clayton DG, Clarke M, Osborne D. Calcaneal ultrasound attenuation in an elderly population: measurement position and relationships with body size and past fractures. Osteoporos Int 1999; 10:316-24.

73. Stewart A, Felsenberg D, Kalidis L, Reid DM. Vertebral fractures in men and women: how discriminative are bone mass measurements? Br J Radiol 1995; 68:614-20.

74. Travers-Gustafson D, Stegman MR, Heaney RP, Recker RR. Ultrasound, densitometry, and extraskeletal appendicular fracture risk factors: a cross-sectional report on the Saunders County Bone Quality Study. Calcif Tissue Int 1995; 57:267-71.

75. Bauer DC, Cauley JA, Ensrud KE, Ewing S, Orwoll ES. Quantitative Ultrasound predicts hip and non-spine fracture in men: the MrOS study. ASBMR 26th Annual Meeting in Seattle, Washington, USA Abstract.

76. Smith MR. Osteoporosis during androgen deprivation therapy for prostate cancer. Urology 2002; 60:79-85; discussion 86.

77. Johnell O, Kanis JA, Oden A, Johansson H, De Laet C, Delmas P, et al. Predictive value of BMD for hip and other fractures. J Bone Miner Res 2005; 20:1185-94.

78. Cummings SR, Cawthon PM, Ensrud KE, Cauley JA, Fink HA, Orwoll ES. BMD and Risk of Hip and Nonvertebral Fractures in Older Men:A Prospective Study and Comparison With Older Women. J Bone Miner Res 2006; 21:1550-6.

79. de Laet CE, van der Klift M, Hofman A, Pols HA. Osteoporosis in men and women: a story about bone mineral density thresholds and hip fracture risk. J Bone Miner Res 2002; 17:2231-6.

80. Melton LJ 3rd, Atkinson EJ, O'Connor MK, O'Fallon WM, Riggs BL. Bone density and fracture risk in men. J Bone Miner Res 1998; 13:1915-23.

81. Faulkner KG, Orwoll E. Implications in the use of T-scores for the diagnosis of osteoporosis in men. J Clin Densitom 2002; 5:87-93.

82. Burgess E, Nanes MS. Osteoporosis in men: pathophysiology, evaluation, and therapy. Curr Opin Rheumatol 2002; 14:421-8.

83. Demirbag D, Ozdemir F, Kokino S, Berkarda S. The relationship between bone mineral density and immobilization duration in hemiplegic limbs. Ann Nucl Med 2005; 19:695-700.

84. Wong SY, Lau EM, Lynn H, Leung PC, Woo J, Cummings SR, et al. Depression and bone mineral density: is there a relationship in elderly Asian men? Results from Mr. Os (Hong Kong). Osteoporos Int 2005; 16:610-5.

85. Sallin U, Mellstrom D, Eggertsen R. Osteoporosis in a nursing home, determined by the DEXA technique. Med Sci Monit 2005; 11:CR67-70.

86. Lim S, Joung H, Shin CS, Lee HK, Kim KS, Shin EK, et al. Body composition changes with age have gender-specific impacts on bone mineral density. Bone 2004; 35:792-8.

87. Reyes MO, Archer JA, Nunlee-Bland G, Daniel G, Morgan OA, Makambi K. Bone mass in physicians: a Howard University Hospital pilot study. J Natl Med Assoc 2004; 96:299-305.

88. Kudlacek S, Schneider B, Peterlik M, Leb G, Klaushofer K, Weber K, et al. Normative data of bone mineral density in an unselected adult Austrian population. Eur J Clin Invest 2003; 33:332-9.

89. Ozdurak RH, Duz S, Arsal G, Akinci Y, Kablan N, Isikli S, et al. Quantitative forearm muscle strength influences radial bone mineral density in osteoporotic and healthy males. Technol Health Care 2003; 11:253-61.

90. Krassas GE, Papadopoulou FG, Doukidis D, Konstantinidis TH, Kalothetou K. Age-related changes in bone density among healthy Greek males. J Endocrinol Invest 2001; 24:326-33.

91. Carr A, Miller J, Eisman JA, Cooper DA. Osteopenia in HIV-infected men: association with asymptomatic lactic acidemia and lower weight pre-antiretroviral therapy. AIDS 2001; 15:703-9.

92. Cetin A, Erturk H, Celiker R, Sivri A, Hascelik Z. The role of quantitative ultrasound in

predicting osteoporosis defined by dual X-ray absorptiometry. Rheumatol Int 2001; 20:55-9.

93. Kemink SA, Hermus AR, Swinkels LM, Lutterman JA, Smals AG. Osteopenia in insulin-dependent diabetes mellitus; prevalence and aspects of pathophysiology. J Endocrinol Invest 2000; 23:295-303.

94. Robinson RJ, al-Azzawi F, Iqbal SJ, Abrams K, Mayberry JF. The relation of hand skin-fold thickness to bone mineral density in patients with Crohn's disease. Eur J Gastroenterol Hepatol 1997; 9:945-9.

95. Cheng S, Suominen H, Sakari-Rantala R, Laukkanen P, Avikainen V, Heikkinen E. Calcaneal bone mineral density predicts fracture occurrence: a five-year follow-up study in elderly people. J Bone Miner Res 1997; 12:1075-82.

96. De Laet CE, Van Hout BA, Burger H, Weel AE, Hofman A, Pols HA. Hip fracture prediction in elderly men and women: validation in the Rotterdam study. J Bone Miner Res 1998; 13:1587-93.

97. Kroger H, Lunt M, Reeve J, Dequeker J, Adams JE, Birkenhager JC, et al. Bone density reduction in various measurement sites in men and women with osteoporotic fractures of spine and hip: the European quantitation of osteoporosis study. Calcif Tissue Int 1999; 64:191-9.

98. Melton LJ 3rd, Beck TJ, Amin S, Khosla S, Achenbach SJ, Oberg AL, et al. Contributions of bone density and structure to fracture risk assessment in men and women. Osteoporos Int 2005; 16:460-7.

99. Odvina CV, Wergedal JE, Libanati CR, Schulz EE, Baylink DJ. Relationship between trabecular vertebral body density and fractures: a quantitative definition of spinal osteoporosis. Metabolism 1988; 37:221-8.

100. Robinson B, Wagstaffe C, Roche J, Clifton-Bligh P, Posen S. Is there a place for forearm osteodensitometry in clinical screening studies? Med J Aust 1987; 146:297-300.

101. Shin MH, Kweon SS, Park KS, Heo H, Kim SJ, Nam HS, et al. Quantitative ultrasound of the calcaneus in a Korean population: reference data and relationship to bone mineral density determined by peripheral dual X-ray absorptiometry. J Korean Med Sci 2005; 20:1011-6.

Appendix A. Data Collection Forms

VA-EPC Male/OP Project Screener

Article ID

Reviewers:
Assigned on:

Citation:

Reviewer: _____

First Author:_____

1. Does the article report original data on the prevalence or incidence of any of the following in men?

(Check all that apply)

Osteopenia ....
Osteoporosis...
Fractures ....
None of the above ....

2. Does the article report original data on risk factors for osteopenia, osteoporosis, or fractures in men?

(Circle one)

Yes..1
No...2

3. Does the article report on a tool to screen for osteoporosis in men?
[tool=radiologic studies, surveys, etc]

(Circle one)

Yes.. 1
No...2

4. Does the article report associations between BMD levels as determined by DXA and fractures in men?

(Circle one)

Yes.. 1
No...2

5. Study design

(Circle one)

RCT/CCT.. 1
Cohort/case series 2
Case control 3
Review article: systematic or M-A 4
Review article: not systematic .... 5 **(STOP)**
Review article: letter, editorial,
other syst review.. 6 **(STOP)**
Other.. 7 **(STOP)**

6. Are any of the subjects identified as veterans?

(Circle one)

Yes.. 1
No.. 2

7. Should this article be saved for background?

(Circle one)

Yes.. 1
No.. 2

NOTES:

VA Male OP Project-Detailed Review Form- Diagnostic Studies

FINAL 09-05-2006

Article ID: _____ Reviewer: _____

First Author: _____
(Last Name Only)

Study Number:
_____ of _____ Description: _____
(Enter '1of 1' if only one) _(if more than one study)_

Do you think that this article might include the same data as another study?
(CIRCLE ONE)

Yes   1
No   2

    If YES enter Trial name and/or IDs:

    Trial name : _____

    ID(s) : _____

What is the study test?

(CHECK ALL THAT APPLY)

Ultrasound, BUA .... ☒
Ultrasound, SOS .... ☒
Ultrasound, QUI .... ☒

Peripheral bone density, pDXA .... ☒
Peripheral bone density, SXA .... ☒
Peripheral bone density, other: _____ ☒

Central DXA .... ☒
Quantitative CT .... ☒
Bone markers .... ☒

Questionnaire, OST .... ☒
Questionnaire, other: _____ ☒

Other: _____ ☒

Other: _____ ☒

If applicable, at what anatomic site was the study test performed?

(CHECK ALL THAT APPLY)

Spine .... ☒
Femur .... ☒
Radius .... ☒

Patella .... ☒
Calcaneus .... ☒
Finger .... ☒

Other: _____ ☒

Not applicable .... ☒
Not reported .... ☒

What is the reference test?

(CHECK ALL THAT APPLY)

Ultrasound, BUA .... ☒
Ultrasound, SOS .... ☒
Ultrasound, QUI .... ☒

Peripheral bone density, pDXA .... ☒
Peripheral bone density, SXA .... ☒
Peripheral bone density, other: _____ ☒

Central DXA .... ☒
Quantitative CT .... ☒

Questionnaire, OST .... ☒
Questionnaire, other: _____ ☒

Prior fractures .... ☒
Prior self-reported osteoporosis .... ☒

Other: _____ ☒

Other: _____ ☒

VA Male OP Project-Detailed Review Form- Diagnostic Studies

If applicable, at what anatomic site was the reference test performed?
(CHECK ALL THAT APPLY)

- Spine ⊠
- Femur ⊠
- Radius ⊠
- Patella ⊠
- Calcaneus ⊠
- Finger ⊠
- Other: _____ ⊠
- Not applicable ⊠
- Not reported ⊠

Who is studied?
(CHECK ALL THAT APPLY)

A. Not reported ⊠
B. Unselected population ⊠
C. Selected population ⊠

Elderly ⊠

- Nursing home ⊠
- Referred ⊠
- Prior glucocorticoid use ⊠
- COPD ⊠
- Hypogonadal ⊠
- Excess alcohol ⊠
- Malabsorption ⊠
- Other: _____

What was the male sample size data? (Enter number or 9999 for not reported)

Enrolled: _____   Followed up: _____

What were the characteristics of the patient population?
(CHECK ALL THAT APPLY)

- Caucasian ⊠
- African Ancestry ⊠
- Hispanic ⊠
- Asian (non-Filipino) ⊠
- Filipino ⊠
- Native American ⊠
- Eskimo/Inuit ⊠
- Other (_____) ⊠
- Veteran ⊠
- Characteristics not reported ⊠

In what region did the study take place?
(CHECK ALL THAT APPLY)

- US/Canada ⊠
- Scandinavia ⊠
- Australia/NZ ⊠
- Western Europe ⊠
- Eastern Europe ⊠
- Latin America ⊠
- Middle East ⊠
- India ⊠
- Africa ⊠
- Asia ⊠
- Other : _____ ⊠
- Not reported ⊠

Does the article report sensitivity, specificity or data to construct 2 X 2 table?
(CHECK ALL THAT APPLY)

- Sensitivity ⊠
- Specificity ⊠
- Correlation ⊠
- Other : _____ ⊠
- Not reported ⊠

VA Male OP QUADAS Quality Review Form

FINAL 10-13-06

Article ID: _____   Reviewer: _____

First Author: _____
(Last Name Only)

Study Number:
_____ of _____ Description: _____
(Enter '1of 1' if only one)   (if more than one study)

1. Was the spectrum of patients representative of the patients who will receive the test in practice?

(CIRCLE ONE)

Yes 1
No 2
Unclear 3

*How to score: Score 'yes' if based on information reported from study's authors, you believe the spectrum of patients included in the study is representative of those in whom the test will be used in practice. Judgment should be based on both method of recruitment and the characteristics of those recruited. Score 'no' if you think the population studied does not fit into what was specified as acceptable. Score 'no' if studies recruit a group of healthy controls and a group known to have the target disorder.

2. Were selection criteria clearly described?

(CIRCLE ONE)

Yes 1
No 2
Unclear 3

*How to score: Score 'yes' if you think all relevant information regarding how participants were selected for inclusion has been provided. Score 'no' if study selection criteria are not clearly reported.

3. Is the reference standard likely to correctly classify the target condition?

(CIRCLE ONE)

Yes 1
No 2
Unclear 3

*How to score: Score 'yes' if you believe the reference standard is likely to correctly classify the target condition or is the best method available. Score 'no' if you do not think the reference standard was likely to have correctly classified the target condition.

4. Is the time period between reference standard and index test short enough to be reasonably sure that the target condition did not change between the two tests?

(CIRCLE ONE)

Yes 1
No 2
Unclear 3

*How to score: For conditions that progress rapidly, should be scored 'yes' if delay between performance of index and ref test if very short. If condition is chronic, longer delay periods may be appropriate. You will have to determine what is 'short enough.' Score 'no' if you think performance of index test and reference standard was sufficiently long that disease status may have changed between the performance of the two tests.

5. Did the whole sample or a random selection of the sample, receive verification using a reference standard?

(CIRCLE ONE)

Yes 1
No 2
Unclear 3

*How to score: Score 'yes' if it is clear that all patients or a random selection of patient who received index test went on to receive verification of disease status using reference standard. Score 'no' if some patients did not receive verification of disease status and selection of patient to receive reference standard was not random.

6. Did patients receive the same reference standard regardless of the index test result?

(CIRCLE ONE)

Yes 1
No 2
Unclear 3

*How to score: Score 'yes' if it is clear that patients received verification of their true disease status using the same reference standard. Score 'no' if some patients received verification using a different reference standard.

VA Male OP QUADAS Quality Review Form

7. Was the reference standard independent of the index test (i.e. the index test did not form part of the reference standard)?

(CIRCLE ONE)

Yes 1
No 2
Unclear 3

*How to score: Score 'yes' if it is clear from the study that the index test did not form part of the reference standard. Score 'no' if it appears that the index test formed part of the reference standard.

8. Was the execution of the index test described in sufficient detail to permit replication of the test?

(CIRCLE ONE)

Yes 1
No 2
Unclear 3

*How to score: SEE # 9

9. Was the execution of the reference standard described in sufficient detail to permit its replication?

(CIRCLE ONE)

Yes 1
No 2
Unclear 3

*How to score: Score 'yes' if study reports sufficient details or citations to permit replication of the index test and reference standard. Score as 'no' in other cases.

10. Were the index test results interpreted without knowledge of the results of the reference standard?

(CIRCLE ONE)

Yes 1
No 2
Unclear 3

*How to score: SEE # 11

11. Were the reference standard results interpreted without knowledge of the results of the index test?

(CIRCLE ONE)

Yes 1
No 2
Unclear 3

*How to score: Score 'yes' if study clearly states that the test results (index or reference standard) were interpreted blind to the results of the other test. Score 'no' if it does not appear that test results were interpreted blind to results of the other test.

12. Were the same clinical data available when test results were interpreted as would be available when the test is used in practice?

(CIRCLE ONE)

Yes 1
No 2
Unclear 3

*How to score: Score 'yes' if clinical data would normally be available when the test is interpreted in practice and similar data were available when interpreting the index test in the study and when clinical data would not be available in practice and these data were not available when the index test results were interpreted. Score 'no' if this is not the case.

13. Were uninterruptible/intermediate test results reported?

(CIRCLE ONE)

Yes 1
No 2
Unclear 3

*How to score: Score 'yes' if it is clear that all test results, including uninterruptible/indeterminate/intermediate results are reported. Score 'no' if you think that such results occurred but have not been reported.

14. Were withdrawals from the study explained?

(CIRCLE ONE)

Yes 1
No 2
Unclear 3

*How to score: Score 'yes' if it is clear what happened to all patients who entered the study, for example if a flow diagram of study participants is reported. Score 'no' if it appears that some of the participants who entered the study did not completed the study (i.e. did not receive both the index test and reference standard and these patients were not accounted for).

VA Male OP Project- RISK FACTOR STUDIES

Article ID: _____   Reviewer: _Elaine Wong_

First Author: _____
(Last Name Only)

Are data in this article reported for MEN for the risk factors listed below?

MODERATE RISK FACTORS
(CHECK ALL THAT APPLY)

Smoking (active) .... ☒
Low Sunlight Exposure (low or none) .... ☒
Family History of Osteoporotic Fracture .... ☒

Low Calcium Intake (<500-850 mg/day) .... ☒
Hyperparathyroidism (N/S) .... ☒
Hyperthyroidism .... ☒

Diabetes mellitus (type II or N/S) .... ☒
Rheumatoid arthritis .... ☒

UNCLASSIFIABLE RISK FACTORS
(CHECK ALL THAT APPLY)

Alcohol Intake.. ☒
Male hypogonadism................................... ☒
Other hormonal factors in men, including

    Anti-androgen therapy .... ☒

Prostaglandin inhibitors (NSAIDs and aspirin) ..... ☒
Anti-ulcer agents .... ☒
Thyroid disease including replacement therapy...... ☒

Respiratory diseases – independent of steroid use .. ☒
Dietary deficiency of Vitamin D................... ☒
Metabolism and GI absorption disorders .... ☒

SCI .... ☒
Hyperhomocysteinemia .... ☒

☒ This article does not include any of the risk factors
listed on this form.

VA Male OP Project-Detailed Review Form- RISK FACTOR STUDIES

FINAL 12/01/06

Article ID: _____ Reviewer: _____

First Author: _____
(Last Name Only)

STUDY PARTICIPATION

	YES	NO
Was the source population clearly defined?..	☒	☒
Was the study population described?.............	☒	
Is the study population representative of the patients of interest (VA)?.............	☒	☒

STUDY DESIGN

4. What is the study design? (Check one)

- Case- Control .... ☒
- Cohort .... ☒
- Cross sectional .... ☒

STUDY ATTRITION

FOR COHORTS ONLY

How many subjects were enrolled?

_____ (ND=9999)

6. How many subjects were included in the data analysis?

_____ (ND=9999)

7. What is the duration of the follow up?

_____ _____
Duration **Units**

OR

_____ person-years

Units
01. Days 04. Years
02. Weeks 05. NR
03. Months

FOR CASE CONTROL ONLY

8. How many cases were included?

_____ _____

9. How many controls were included?

_____ _____

FOR CROSS SECTIONAL STUDIES ONLY

10. What is the sample size?

_____ _____

RISRIRISK FACTOR MEASUREMENT

Which of the following risk factors were assessed?

Alcohol Consumption .... ☒
- If yes, how was alcohol consumption defined:

_____

Diabetes Mellitus, type II or NOS .... ☒
- If yes, how was the presence of diabetes defined:

_____

Spinal Cord Injury... ☒
- If yes, how was the presence and location of SCI defined:

_____

VA Male OP Project-Detailed Review Form- RISK FACTOR STUDIES

OUTCOME MEASUREMENT

12. What outcome was assessed?

BMD (cDXA).. ☒

If yes answer the following: (CHECK ALL THAT APPLY)

- Site
  - Spine .... ☒
  - Femur .... ☒
  - Radius .... ☒

  - Patella...................................... ☒
  - Calcaneus................................. ☒
  - Finger .... ☒
  - Other: _____ .... ☒

  - Not applicable .... ☒
  - Not reported .... ☒

- T-score: _____

- Reference Standard
  - Male .... ☒
  - Female..................................... ☒
  - Other .... ☒

  Specify: _____

Osteoporotic fracture.. ☒

If yes, how was the presence of fracture assessed: (CHECK ALL THAT APPLY)

- X-ray .... ☒
- Diary/Self Report .... ☒
- Administrative data..................... ☒
- Medical Record Review............... ☒

Other Bone Measurements................................... ☒

If yes, please specify: (CHECK ALL THAT APPLY)

- Ultrasound................................. ☒
- Other .... ☒

Specify: _____

POTEPOTENTIAL CONFOUNDING PROGNOSTIC FACTOR MEASUREMENT

13. Which of the following risk factors were assessed?

(CHECK ALL THAT APPLY)

- Age.. ☒
- Low body weight .... ☒
- Weight loss................................. ☒

- Physical inactivity/prolonged immobilization
  (Not SCI)................................. ☒
- Corticosteroid use .... ☒
- Anticonvulsant use .... ☒

- Hyperparathyroidism .... ☒
- Diabetes Mellitus, type I .... ☒
- Gastrectomy................................ ☒

- Hypogonadism, primary or secondary ...... ☒
- Poor visual acuity........................ ☒
- Previous osteoporotic fracture ...... ☒

- Cigarette smoking........................ ☒
- Vitamin D deficiency................... ☒
- Low dietary calcium intake........... ☒

- Family History of Osteoporotic Fracture ...... ☒
- Hyperthyroidism.......................... ☒
- Rheumatoid Arthritis.................... ☒
- High bone turnover rate .... ☒

ANALANALYSIS

14. Does the article present: (CHECK THAT APPLY)

- Bivariate.................................... ☒
- Multivariate................................ ☒
- Other .... ☒

Specify: _____

VA Male OP Project – RISK FACTOR STUDIES, Quality Measurement

Article ID: _____   Reviewer: _____

First Author: _____
(Last Name Only)

STUDY PARTICIPATION

The study sample represents the population of interest on key characteristics, sufficient to limit potential bias to the results.

Yes.................... ☒
Partly.................... ☒
No.................... ☒
Unsure.................... ☒

*Population of interest is adequately described for key characteristics
*Sampling frame and recruitment are adequately described, including methods to identity the sample (number and type used, e.g., referral patterns in health care), period of recruitment, and place of recruitment (setting and geographic location).
*Inclusion and exclusion criteria are adequately described (e.g., including explicit diagnostic criteria or "zero time" description).
* There is adequate participation in the study by eligible individuals.
*The baseline study sample (i.e., individuals entering the study) is adequately described for key characteristics.

STUDY ATTRITION

Loss to follow-up (from sample to study population) is not associated with key characteristics (i.e., the study data adequately represent the sample), sufficient to limit potential bias.

Yes.................... ☒
Partly.................... ☒
No.................... ☒
Unsure.................... ☒

*Proportion of study sample completing the study and providing outcome data is adequate.
*Attempts to collect information on participants who dropped out of the study are described.
*Reasons for loss to follow-up are provided.
*Participants lost to follow-up are adequately described for key characteristics.
*There are no important differences between key characteristics and outcomes in participants who completed the study and those who did not.

PROGPROGNOSTIC FACTOR MEASUREMENT

The prognostic factor of interest is adequately measured in study participants to sufficiently limit potential bias.

Yes.................... ☒
Partly.................... ☒
No.................... ☒
Unsure.................... ☒

*A clear definition or description of the prognostic factor measure is provided (e.g., including dose, level, duration of exposure, and clear specification of the method of measurement.)
*Continuous variables are reported or appropriate (i.e., not data-dependent) cut-points are used.
*The prognostic factor measure and method are adequately valid and reliable to limit misclassification Bias (e.g. may include relevant outside sources of information on measurement properties, also characteristics, such as blind measurement and limited reliance on recall).
*Adequate proportion of the study sample has complete data for prognostic factors.
*The method and setting of measurement are the same for all study participants.
*Appropriate methods are used if imputation is used for missing prognostic factor data.

OUTCOME MEASUREMENT

The outcome of interest is adequately measured in study participants to sufficiently limit potential bias.

Yes.................... ☒
Partly.................... ☒
No.................... ☒
Unsure.................... ☒

*A clear definition of the outcome of interest is provided, including duration of follow-up and level and extent of the outcome construct.
*The outcome measure and method used are adequately valid and reliable to limit misclassification bias (e.g., may include relevant outside sources of information on measurement properties, also characteristics, such as blind measurement and confirmation of outcome with valid and reliable test.)
*The method and setting of measurement are the same for all study participants.

VA Male OP Project – RISK FACTOR STUDIES, Quality Measurement

CONFOUNDING MEASUREMENT AND ACCOUNT

Important potential confounders are appropriately accounted for, limiting potential bias with respect to the prognostic factor of interest.

Yes .... ☐
Partly .... ☐
No .... ☐
Unsure .... ☐

*All important confounders, including treatments (key variables in conceptual model), are measured.
*Clear definitions of the important confounders measured are provided (e.g., including dose, level and duration of exposures).
*Measurement of all important confounders is adequately valid and reliable (e.g., may include relevant outside sources of information on measurement properties, also characteristics, such as blind measurement and limited reliance on recall.)
*The method and setting of confounding measurement are the same for all study participants.
*Appropriate methods are used if imputation is used for missing confounder data.
*Important potential confounders are accounted for in the study design (e.g., matching for key variables, stratification, or initial assembly of comparable groups.)
*Important potential confounders are accounted for in the analysis (i.e., appropriate adjustment).

ANALYSIS

The statistical analysis is appropriate for the design of the study, limiting potential for presentation of invalid results.

Yes .... ☐
Partly .... ☐
No .... ☐
Unsure .... ☐

*There is sufficient presentation of data to assess the adequacy of the analysis.
*The strategy for model building (i.e., inclusion of variables) is appropriate and is based on a conceptual framework or model.
* The selected model is adequate for the design of the study.
*There is no selective reporting of results.

Appendix B. Evidence Table

Evidence Table 1. Diagnostic Test Studies
Columns 1-10: Article, Population, Characteristics, Sample Size, Study test & site, Reference test & site, QUADAS, Results

Author, Year, Region, Trial Name	Population	Characteristics	Male sample size	Study Test	Study Site	Reference Test	Reference Site	QUADAS*	Results
Adler, 2001 [27] US/Canada	Referred for DXA	NR, Veteran	185	Ultrasound BUA & QUI	Calcaneus	Central DXA	Spine, Femur	3,3,1,1,1,1, 1,1,3,3,1,1,3	**Central DXA T-score<-1.5** Heel T-score=0: Sens=0.89, Spec=0.40 Heel T-score<-0.5: Sens=0.79, Spec=0.48 Heel T-score<-1.0: Sens=0.65, Spec=0.75 Heel T-score<-1.5: Sens=0.49, Spec=0.84 Heel T-score<-2.0: Sens=0.30, Spec=0.94 Heel T-score<-2.5: Sens=0.07, Spec=0.98 **Central DXA T-score<-2.0** Heel T-score=0: Sens=0.92, Spec=0.35 Heel T-score<-0.5: Sens=0.86, Spec=0.47 Heel T-score<-1.0: Sens=0.71, Spec=0.68 Heel T-score<-1.5: Sens=0.53, Spec=079 Heel T-score<-2.0: Sens=0.30, Spec=0.89 Heel T-score<-2.5: Sens=0.06, Spec=0.97 **Central DXA T-score<-2.5** Heel T-score=0: Sens=0.91, Spec=0.27 Heel T-score<-0.5: Sens=0.86, Spec=0.38 Heel T-score<-1.0: Sens=0.74, Spec=0.59 Heel T-score<-1.5: Sens=0.60, Spec=0.73 Heel T-score<-2.0: Sens=0.34, Spec=0.86 Heel T-score<-2.5: Sens=0.07, Spec=0.97
Adler, 2003 [19] US/Canada	Pulmonary Clinic	Asian, Veteran	107	Ultrasound BUA, SOS & QUI; questionnaire	Calcaneus	Central DXA	Spine, Femur	1,1,1,1,2,1,1, 1,1,3,3,1,1,3	Central DXA T-score<-2.0, Heel T-score<-1.5: Sens=0.41, Spec=0.77
Adler, 2003 [35] US/Canada	Pulmonary & Rheumatology Clinic	Pulmonary & Rheumatology Clinic, Veteran	181	Questionnaire OST	NA	Central DXA	Spine, Femur	1,1,1,1,1,1,1, 1,3,3,1,1,1	**Central DXA T-score<-2.0** OSTA score<1: Sens=0.62, Spec=0.89 OSTA score<2: Sens=0.69, Spec=0.82 OSTA score<3: Sens=0.74, Spec=0.72 **Central DXA T-score<-2.5** OSTA score<1: Sens=0.75, Spec=0.80 OSTA score<2: Sens=0.82, Spec=0.74 OSTA score<3: Sens=0.93, Spec=0.66
Cheng, 1997 [95] Scandinavia	Elderly	NR	205	Peripheral bone density pDXA	Calcaneus	Fracture Occurrence	Multiple Sites	2,1,1,2,1,1, 1,1,3,3,1,1,1	Determined that calcaneal BMD can be used as a predictor of fracture occurrence in 75-80 year old men.
De Laet, 1998 [96] Western Europe	Elderly	NR	2778	Central DXA, Hiefy Risk using DCA	Femur, NA	Fracture Occurrence	NA	1,1,1,1,1,1,1, 1,3,3,1,1,1	Evaluated a hip fracture risk equation which included age and femoral neck BMD and found that they were able to accurately predict hip fracture over an approximate four year period.
Donaldson, 1999 [72] Western Europe	Elderly	NR	817	Ultrasound BUA	Calcaneus	Fracture Occurrence	NR	1,1,3,1,2,3,1, 1,1,3,3,1,1,2	Found no significant difference between fixed or anatomic BUA values in men with or without a past fracture.

*QUADAS 1=Yes, 2=No, 3=Unclear; Order is: Spectrum representativeness, Selection criteria, Reference standard, Time period, Verification bias, Use of same reference test, Independence, Detail of index test, Details of reference test, Blinding #1, Blinding #2, Usefulness in practice, Intermediate results, Withdrawls

NR=Not Reported
SOS=Speed of sound
SI=Stiffness Index

BUA=Broad-band ultrasound attenuation
OST=Osteoporosis Screening Tool
OSTA=Osteoporosis Screening Tool for Asians

QUI=Quantitative Ultrasound Index
BMD=Bone Mass Density
MOST=Male Osteoporosis Screening Tool

DXA=Dual energy x-ray absorptiometry
QUS=Quantitative Ultrasound
AVU=Apparent velocity of ultrasound

Evidence Table 1. Diagnostic Test Studies
Columns 1-10: Article, Population, Characteristics, Sample Size, Study test & site, Reference test & site, QUADAS, Results

Author, Year, Region,	Population	Characteristics	Male sample size	Study Test	Study Site	Reference Test	Reference Site	QUADAS*	Results
Gonnelli, 2005 [68] Western Europe	Bone Clinic	NR	407	Ultrasound BUA & SOS; Central DXA	Spine, Femur, Calcaneus	Fracture Occurrence	Spine, Femur, Radius, Pelvis	2,1,1,1,1,1, 1,1,3,3,1,1	Found that hip BMD (OR 3.4, 2.5-4.8) and QUS stiffness (OR 3.2, 2.3-4.5) had strong associations with fractures and that combining these two parameters resulted in an even stronger association (OR 6.1, 2.6-14.3).
Grampp, 2001 [66] Western Europe	Referred for BMD	NR	501	Ultrasound QUS	Calcaneus	Central DXA	Spine, Femur	2,1,1,1,1,1, 1,1,3,3,1,1	Insufficient statistics for sensitivity and specificity calculation
Gudmundsdottir, 2005 [20] Scandinavia	Unselected	NR	589	Ultrasound BUA, SOS & SI	Calcaneus	Central DXA	Spine, Femur	2,1,1,3,1,1, 1,1,3,3,1,2	**Total hip DXA T-score<-2.5** QUS T-score<0: Sens=1.0, Spec=0.14 QUS T-score<-0.5: Sens=0.86, Spec=0.28 QUS T-score<-1.0: Sens=0.82, Spec=0.49 **Femoral neck BMD T-score<-2.5** QUS T-score<0: Sens=1.0, Spec=0.13 QUS T-score<-0.5: Sens=0.92, Spec=0.28 QUS T-score<-1.0: Sens=0.83, Spec=0.47
Kaptoge, 2004 [17] Western Europe	Unselected	NR	2653	Simple Score Male Multivariate Model	Spine	Fracture Occurrence	Spine, Femur, Radius, Rib, Other	1,1,1,1,1,1, 1,1,3,3,1,1	Found that the risk for prevalent vertebral fracture significantly increased with age (RR 1.3, 1.2-1.5), height loss (RR 1.1, 1.0-1.1), self-reported spine fractures (RR 5.1, 3.7-6.9), and weight (RR 0.9, 0.8-0.9).
Karlsson, 1996 [14] Scandinavia	Unselected	NR	33	Central DXA; X-ray	Femur	Fracture Occurrence	Femur	1,1,1,1,1,1, 1,1,3,3,1,1	Found a significant correlation between age and femoral shaft width (r=0.4), cervical width (r=0.4); no significant correlation was found between radiographic signs of osteoporosis and DXA hip values.
Kroger, 1999 [97] Scandinavia, Western Europe	Referred – PCP	NR	68	Central DXA; Quantitative CT	Spine, Femur	Fracture Occurrence	Spine, Femur	3,2,1,3,3,3,1, 1,1,3,3,3,3	Found that axial and peripheral quantitative CT performed comparably to DXA in spinal osteoporosis assessment.
Kung, 2005 [63] Asia	Elderly	Asian	776	Ultrasound BUA; SOS & QUI; OSTA	Calcaneus NA	Central DXA	Spine, Femur	2,1,1,1,1,1, 1,1,3,3,1,3	**Femoral neck BMD T-score<-2.5** OSTA score <-1.0: Sens=0.71, Spec=0.68 QUI T-score<-1.2: Sens=0.76, Spec=0.72
Li-Yu, 2005 [15] Asia	Unselected	Filipino	132	OSTA	NA	Central DXA	Femur	2,1,1,1,1,1, 2,3,1,1,3,3	**Femoral neck BMD T-score<-2.5** OSTA score <-1.0: Sens=0.91, Spec=0.66
Lynn, 2005 [65] Asia	Elderly	Asian	2000	Ultrasound QUI; MOST	NA	Central DXA	Spine, Femur	2,1,1,1,3,1,1, 1,1,3,3,1,1	**Central BMD T-score <-2.5** MOST score > 3: Sens=0.94, Spec=0.46
Melton, 2005 [98] US/Canada	Unselected	NR	348	Bone Structural Parameters	Femur	Central DXA, Fracture Occurrence	Femur	1,1,1,1,1,2, 1,1,3,3,1,2	Found that the best predictors of osteoporotic fractures in a multivariate in men included age (OR per 10 years, 1.5; 1.1-2.1), femoral neck section modulus (OR, 1.6; 1.1-2.5), and intertrochanteric buckling ratio (OR 1.6; 1.3-2.0).
Montagnani, 2001 [67] Western Europe	Unselected	NR	182	Central DXA; Ultrasound	Spine, Femur, Finger	Fracture Occurrence	NR	1,2,1,1,1,1, 1,1,3,3,1,1	Evaluated usefulness of ultrasound of the phalanx and in regression analysis found that only one parameter, bone transmission time (BTT), was comparable to DXA parameters in determining fracture risk.

*QUADAS 1=Yes, 2=No, 3=Unclear; Order is: Spectrum representativeness, Selection criteria, Reference standard, Time period, Verification bias, Use of same reference test, Independence, Detail of index test, Details of reference test, Blinding #1, Blinding #2, Usefulness in practice, Intermediate results, Withdrawls

NR=Not Reported   BUA=Broad-band ultrasound attenuation   QUI=Quantitative Ultrasound Index   DXA=Dual energy x-ray absorptiometry
SOS=Speed of sound   OST=Osteoporosis Screening Tool   BMD=Bone Mass Density   QUS=Quantitative Ultrasound
SI=Stiffness Index   OSTA=Osteoporosis Screening Tool for Asians   MOST=Male Osteoporosis Screening Tool   AVU=Apparent velocity of ultrasound

Evidence Table 1. Diagnostic Test Studies
Columns 1-10: Article, Population, Characteristics, Sample Size, Study test & site, Reference test & site, QUADAS, Results

Author, Year, Region,	Population	Characteristics	Male sample size	Study		Reference		QUADAS*	Results
				Test	Site	Test	Site		
Mulleman, 2002 [#1274] Western Europe	Referral	NR	102	Ultrasound BUA, SOS & SI	Calcaneus	Central DXA, Fracture Occurrence	Spine, Femur	2,1,3,1,1,1,1,1,3,3,1,1,1	Quantitative ultrasound (QUS) is associated with low-trauma fracture (OR 2.3 and 2.1 for SOS and SI respectively), although sensitivity is less than when results are compared with BMD at the lumbar spine (OR 2.8) and hip (OR=3.4) with an area under the curve in ROC analysis for BMD of Lumbar spine = 0.80 and BUA 0.69 (P<0.05). **Lumbar spine DXA T-score<=-2.5** QUS T-score <=-2.5: Sens=0.56, Spec=0.84; **Femoral neck DXA T-score<=-2.5** QUS T-score <=-2.5: Sens=0.64, Spec=0.74; **Hip DXA T-score<=-2.5** QUS T-score <=-2.5: Sens=0.41, Spec=0.93; **Stiffness index DXA T-score <=-2.5** QUS T-score <=-2.5: Sens=0.60, Spec=0.78;
Odvina, 1988 [99] US/Canada	Referral for Osteoporosis	NR, Veteran	38	Quantitative CT	Spine	Fracture Occurrence		2,1,1,1,1,1,1,1,3,3,1,1,1	Employed trabecular vertebral body density by CT to determine fracture threshold in men and women. Although fracture threshold was not well defined in men, the values obtained by different methods were in close agreement to those noted in women. Fracture threshold was higher in men than women (123 ±7 vs. 101 ±2 mg/cm³, p<0.001).
Robinson, 1987 [100] Australia	Referred by Hospital Staff	NR	31	Linear Photon Absorptiometry	Spine, Radius	Quantitative CT, Fracture Occurrence	Spine	2,2,1,1,3,3,1,1,3,3,1,1,3	Found that men with vertebral fractures has significantly lower mean forearm osteodensitometry and spinal mineral content than age matched men without a history of fractures (16 point difference in "arbitrary units," p<0.02; 65 mg equivalent K²HPO₄/cm³, p<0.0025, respectively).
Rothenberg, 2004 [70] US/Canada	Unselected	NR	301	Ultrasound Bone Density	Calcaneus	Fracture Occurrence	Spine, Femur, Radius, Shoulder, Ribs	1,1,3,1,1,1,1,1,3,3,1,1,1	Estimated that the Hologic T-score of -0.2 corresponds to a BMD of 0.57 gm/cm² which corresponds to an increase in relative risk of fracture of 1.4.
Shin, 2005 [101] Asia	Unselected, Elderly	Asian	1225	Ultrasound BUA, SOS & Stiffness	Calcaneus	Peripheral bone density pDXA	Radius, Calcaneus	2,1,1,1,1,1,1,1,3,3,1,1,2	Found that correlations between QUS and BMD were 0.41 to 0.73 in men, with peak mean values for QUS occurring in men aged 20-29 years old.
Stewart, 1995 [73] Western Europe	Unselected	NR	247	Ultrasound BUA; Central DXA	Spine, Femur, Calcaneus	Fracture Occurrence	Spine	1,3,1,1,1,1,1,1,3,3,1,1,1	No statistically significant relationship between BUA or DXA at any site and fractures in men in bivariate analyses.
Travers-Gustafson, 1995 [74] US/Canada	Elderly	NR	529	Peripheral Bone Density other; AVU	Radius, Patella	Fracture Occurrence	NR	1,1,3,1,1,1,1,1,3,3,1,1,1	Apparent velocity of ultrasound (AVU) is highly associated with low trauma fractures in both women (OR 1.46, 95% CI=1.18,1.81) and men (OR 1.69, 95% CI=1.24,2.32).

*QUADAS 1=Yes, 2=No, 3=Unclear; Order is: Spectrum representativeness, Selection criteria, Reference standard, Time period, Verification bias, Use of same reference test, Independence, Detail of index test, Details of reference test, Blinding #1, Blinding #2, Usefulness in practice, Intermediate results, Withdrawls

NR=Not Reported
SOS=Speed of sound
SI=Stiffness Index

BUA=Broad-band ultrasound attenuation
OST=Osteoporosis Screening Tool
OSTA=Osteoporosis Screening Tool for Asians

QUI=Quantitative Ultrasound Index
BMD=Bone Mass Density
MOST=Male Osteoporosis Screening Tool

DXA=Dual energy x-ray absorptiometry
QUS=Quantitative Ultrasound
AVU=Apparent velocity of ultrasound

Evidence Table 1. Diagnostic Test Studies

Columns 1-10: Article, Population, Characteristics, Sample Size, Study test & site, Reference test & site, QUADAS, Results

Author, Year, Region,	Population	Characteristics	Male sample size	Study		Reference		QUADAS[*]	Results
				Test	Site	Test	Site		
Varenna, 2005 [69] Western Europe	Unselected	NR	4832	Ultrasound BUA, SOS, & SI	Calcaneus	Fracture Occurrence	Femur, Non-spinal	1,1,3,1,1,1,1, 1,1,3,3,1,1,1	Found that each SD reduction in QUS measurement resulted in a significant approximate 2X increase in risk of hip fracture, independent of age and other clinical variables, consistent with findings found in elderly women.
Welch, 2004 [71] Western Europe	Unselected	NR	6860	Ultrasound BUA	Calcaneus	Fracture Occurrence	Spine, Femur, Radius	1,1,3,1,1,1,1, 1,1,3,3,1,1,1	Found differences sex differences in relationship between osteoporosis risk factors and BUA. Age, weight, and height explained 27% of the variance of BUA in women, but only 3% in men.
Bauer, 2006 [75] US/Canada	Elderly	NR	5608	Ultrasound BUA, Central DXA	Femur, Calcaneus	Fracture Occurrence	Femur	1,1,1,1,1,1,1, 3,3,1,1,1,1,3	Each SD decrease in calcaneal ultrasound BUA was associated with an increased rate of hip (RH= 1.97, CI: 1.32, 3.54) and non-spine (RH=1.65, CI: 1.38,1.96) fracture. Ultrasound predicted hip and non-spine fractures almost as well as femoral BMD, and the combination of these tests was not better than either test alone.

[*]QUADAS 1=Yes, 2=No, 3=Unclear; Order is: Spectrum representativeness, Selection criteria, Reference standard, Time period, Verification bias, Use of same reference test, Independence, Detail of index test, Details of reference test, Blinding #1, Blinding #2, Usefulness in practice, Intermediate results, Withdrawls

NR=Not Reported
SOS=Speed of sound
SI=Stiffness Index

BUA=Broad-band ultrasound attenuation
OST=Osteoporosis Screening Tool
OSTA=Osteoporosis Screening Tool for Asians

QUI=Quantitative Ultrasound Index
BMD=Bone Mass Density
MOST=Male Osteoporosis Screening Tool

DXA=Dual energy x-ray absorptiometry
QUS=Quantitative Ultrasound
AVU=Apparent velocity of ultrasound